NUTRITION IN MOTHER AND CHILD HEALTH

Macmillan Tropical Community Health Manuals
General Editor: Dr J. Grant, London School of Hygiene and Tropical Medicine

This series has been set up specifically to meet the needs of trainee and practising medical personnel in the tropical and sub-tropical developing countries. Some of the books will appeal to others involved in Community work — e.g. school teachers, public health inspectors, environmental health officers, and even literate parents. Early on there will be heavy concentration on aspects of care offering best prospects for improved standards of preventative treatment and therefore health in the community. Inevitably there will be strong emphasis on infant, child and mother care, as infants and children account for up to half the total population in some tropical developing countries, and more than half of the presentations for treatment.

Most titles will be short practical books written for trainee and practising doctors, nurses, auxiliaries, medical officers and assistants and other grades of health-care personnel engaged in frontline health-care delivery, often in small rural centres and sub-centres.

Other titles by G. J. Ebrahim in the Macmillan Tropical Community Health Manuals Series

Child Care in the Tropics	cased	ISBN 0 333 24038 3
	paper	ISBN 0 333 25361 2
Handbook of Tropical Paediatrics	cased	ISBN 0 333 24039 1
	paper	ISBN 0 333 25364 7
Practical Mother and Child Health in Developing Countries	cased	ISBN 0 333 24111 8
	paper	ISBN 0 333 25363 9
Care of the Newborn in Developing Countries	cased	ISBN 0 333 24112 6
	paper	ISBN 0 333 25362 0
Breast Feeding: the Biological Option	cased	ISBN 0 333 23802 8
	paper	ISBN 0 333 23803 6

The paperback edition of this book is available at a reduced price for use in developing countries. This has been made possible by a generous subsidy provided by the Catholic Fund for Overseas Development, 2 Garden Close, Stockwell Road, London, SW9 9TY. CAFOD have also provided subsidies for the production of reduced price editions of other books in the series. The publishers and authors would like to acknowledge the valuable role of CAFOD in this respect.

NUTRITION IN MOTHER AND CHILD HEALTH

G J EBRAHIM

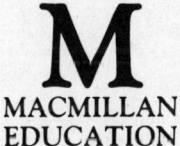
MACMILLAN
EDUCATION

Published with the support of the Catholic Fund for Overseas Development

© G. J. Ebrahim 1983

All rights reserved. No reproduction, copy or transmission of this publication may be made without written permission.

No paragraph of this publication may be reproduced, copied or transmitted save with written permission or in accordance with the provisions of the Copyright Act 1956 (as amended), or under the terms of any licence permitting limited copying issued by the Copyright Licensing Agency, 7 Ridgmount Street, London WC1E 7AE.

Any person who does any unauthorised act in relation to this publication may be liable to criminal prosecution and civil claims for damages.

First published 1983
Reprinted 1987

Published by
MACMILLAN EDUCATION LTD
Houndmills, Basingstoke, Hampshire RG21 2XS
and London
Companies and representatives
throughout the world

Printed in Hong Kong

ISBN 0-333-26965-9 (hardcover)
ISBN 0-333-26966-7 (paperback)

CONTENTS

1 **Introduction**   1
   Systems through which man interacts with environment to obtain food − Further reading

2 **Common Tropical Foods**   16
   The major cereals − Tubers and fruits used as staple foods − Legumes − Edible oil plants − Milk and milk products − Preparing a balanced diet from locally available foods − Further reading

3 **Nutrition in Pregnancy and the Growth of the Fetus**   34
   Effects of the previous health and nutritional status of the mother − Fetal growth − Nutritional requirements of the fetus − The role of the placenta − Mechanism of placental transfer − Nutrition of the mother − Cellular growth in the fetus − Weight at birth and body composition of the fetus − Effects of supplementing maternal diet − Intervention programmes − Further reading

4 **Breast Feeding**   54
   Protein requirements − Human milk as a nutrient − Dangers of artificial feeding − Human milk as a protective agent − Biological mediator: a new role for breast milk − Mother-infant relationship − The spacing of pregnancies − Intervention programmes − Interventions at the community level − Interventions at the national level − Further reading

5 **The Weaning Period**   83
   Dangers of the weaning period − Traditional dietary practices resulting in low intake of energy − Food intake and appetite in the weanling − The role of intercurrent infections − Catch-up growth − Longitudinal studies − The role of infection in the aetiology of malnutrition − Gut dynamics in malnutrition − Intervention programmes − Food production: policies and constraints − The question of bulk in the weaning diet − Prevention of contamination − Provision of health services − Part-time village health workers − Further reading

6   **Protein-Energy Malnutrition**   104
    Classification and definition – Clinical features – Associated deficiencies – Pathological features and changes in metabolism – Management – Innovative approaches – Community-centred approaches – Monitoring the nutrition of the community – Further reading

7   **Vitamins in Health and Disease**   134
    Vitamin A and xerophthalmia – Rickets and metabolic bone disease – Deficiencies of vitamins of the B group – Summary – Further reading

8   **Nutritional Anaemias**   167
    Prevalence – Aetiological factors – Further reading

9   **Community Programmes for Better Nutrition**   182
    The need for a district inventory of nutrition interventions – Coverage, a key issue – Estimating target groups – The need for integration – Innovative approaches – The three tiers in the iceberg of malnutrition – A strategy of 'nutrition with the people' – Urban areas – Further reading

    Index   196

Preface

Within the first few days of commencing work as a paediatrician in Tanzania I came to appreciate the important role of nutrition in child health. Fully half the number of children in the paediatric wards on an average day had illnesses related to malnutrition in one way or another, and yet my training had not prepared me adequately for its prevention in the community. The teaching of nutrition in my days was largely part of the physiological sciences, especially biochemistry. In the classical medical curriculum nutritional disorders are mainly taught as biochemical deficiencies of essential nutrients resulting in typical physiological changes which present as clinical symptoms and signs. The social, cultural and economic aspects of feeding the individual members of the family are rarely discussed. Malnutrition is considered to stem largely from ignorance. Consequently a great deal of effort is put into nutrition education both in the hospital and in the community. This classical approach must be questioned, largely because in most countries there has been no impact on the prevalence of malnutrition despite heavy investment in training programmes and in nutrition education.

If malnutrition is due to ignorance, then how is it that a large number of parents in traditional societies are able to bring up healthy children? Such questioning has led to the identification of the important role of infection in the etiology of nutritional disorders. In communities where the common infectious illnesses of childhood have been adequately controlled by immunisation, and where facilities exist for oral rehydration, childhood malnutrition has been minimised. Such observations provide the basis for integrating nutrition activities with health programmes. Secondly, malnutrition has come to be recognised as part of the spectrum of the disadvantages of poverty. At first glance health workers may feel helpless in the face of this formidable problem; and yet in several projects around the world, committed individuals have evolved approaches to deal with the challenge of poverty. Reference is made to these approaches in several chapters and in the final chapter a total community approach is described based on my experience in Tanzania.

In the peasant society, food production largely determines the state of nutrition of the individual. Urban growth is dependent on rural areas for food supply. In several countries agricultural productivity has not kept pace with developments in other sectors, with the result that an increasing number of previously food-exporting countries have become net importers. This makes them economically and politically vulnerable. It also exposes their populations to newer foods and to exploitation by the food processing industry. Valuable national food resources may not be adequately utilised. A good example is that of human milk and the marked decline in breast feeding in many countries with tragic consequences.

Several friends and colleagues have influenced my own thinking and approach to nutrition in the developing world. In particular my association with David Morley has made me appreciate the need for low cost innovative approaches. The Under-5s Clinic and the Road to Health Chart are but two examples of such approaches. In many communities where these two concepts have been correctly applied, there has been a rapid decline in childhood malnutrition.

Finally, the book is part of a system of texts and, for reasons of economy, concepts and activities described in one book are not repeated in another. Thus, the Under-5s Clinic is described in "Practical Mother and Child Health in Developing Countries" and the weight chart has been discussed in "Paediatric Practice in Developing Countries". After a great deal of thought, and consultations with several colleagues, it was felt that duplication was to be avoided to keep production costs down. All the titles in the series, including the present one, have been produced at a specially low price for the developing world. The continuing support of CAFOD (Catholic Fund for Overseas Development) and the co-operation of the publishers have helped in achieving this aim and are gratefully acknowledged.

G J Ebrahim

Chapter 1

Introduction

Man needs food to provide energy for the body's essential physiological functions like respiration, circulation, digestion and metabolism; for maintaining body temperature; for the growth and repair of the body's tissues; and for obtaining essential nutrients which perform key functions in the biochemical processes of metabolism. The food that man eats is vegetable or animal in origin, and in both forms the energy which it provides is basically solar energy which has been 'trapped' by photosynthesis and stored in various organs of the plant. Man, in common with other species of the animal kingdom, obtains this energy either by consuming these parts of the plant, e.g. cereal or tuber, or secondarily by consuming animals which live on plants, or their products.

In common with all living organisms, man obtains food by interaction with his environment. Prior to the development of agriculture man was a hunter-gatherer and ate what his environment provided. Several tribes in Africa, the aborigines of Australia, and the Eskimo are still by and large in this stage of development and their means of obtaining food from the environment can be described by the model in figure 1.1. With the beginning of agriculture, man evolved agricultural technology, social systems and cultural practices to enable him to interact with his environment singly or in groups in order to obtain a regular

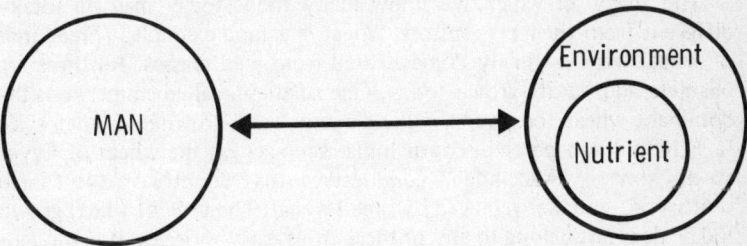

Figure 1.1   Obtaining nutrients from the environment – the hunter-gatherer stage

supply of food. Commerce and marketing has also been part of this development and in recent years this aspect of food production has grown into 'agribusiness' which is concerned with the processing, sale and marketing of foods in different forms on national and even global scales. This aspect of man's interaction with his environment is demonstrated by the model in figure 1.2.

Figure 1.2   Obtaining nutrients from the environment − the complex society

From the beginning of the practice of agriculture there has been a tendency to concentrate on those species of plants that are most productive and rewarding in terms of labour (and capital) invested. In the past few centuries this trend has accelerated, especially with the coming of industrialisation and the development of cash economies. Supermarkets and convenience foods have further restricted choice in diets in urban industrial societies and through the development of multinational corporations are exerting their influence on Third World countries as well. This trend for more and more people to be nourished by fewer varieties of plants has reached the stage where a large proportion of the world's population is dependent on a handful of plant species. Four crops − wheat, rice, maize and potato − together contribute more to the world food supply than all the other crops put together. Figures 1.3−1.5 show the main parts of the world where the common food crops are raised.

The forms in which we know many foods today may be totally different from their progenitors. Wheat is a good example. Three kinds of wheat were originally domesticated from wild grasses. All three are obsolete and hardly grown today. One of these, called emmer, was the dominant wheat for several millennia and is still grown on a small scale in Ethiopia and parts of south India. Emmer was the wheat of Egypt at the time of Alexander's conquest of that country in the fourth century BC and was replaced by bread wheat. The type of wheat grown today does not belong to any of these three early varieties. It is thought that a mutated form of emmer is the ancestor of the common 'macaroni wheat' and that hybridisation with a wild goat-grass gave rise to a form

Introduction

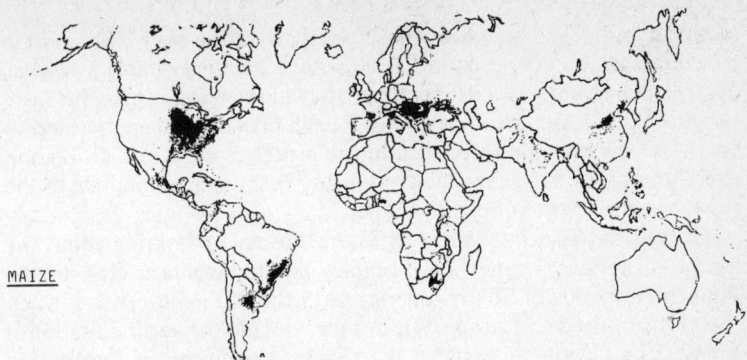

Figure 1.3   Principal sources of maize (total world output: 300 million tonnes)

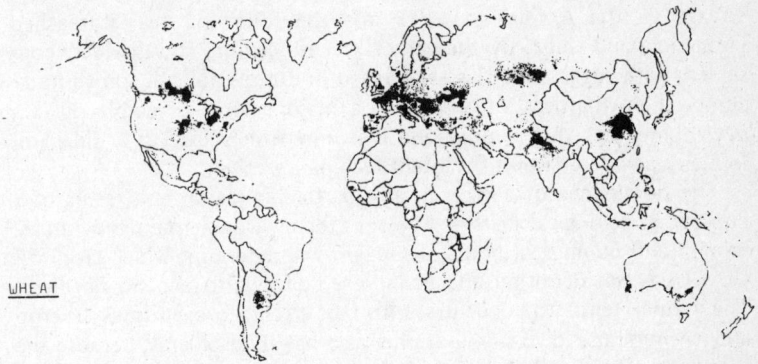

Figure 1.4   Principal sources of wheat (total world output: 350 million tonnes)

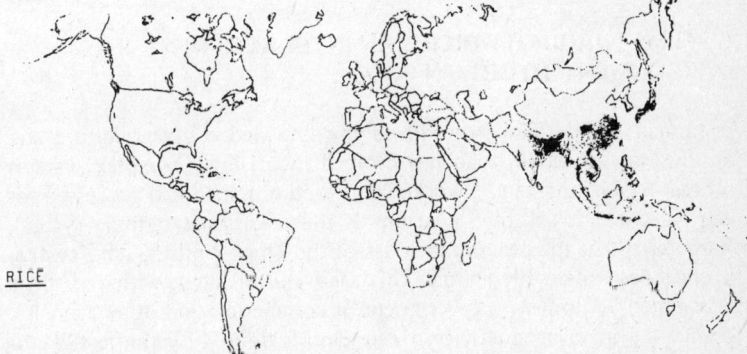

Figure 1.5   Principal sources of rice (total world output: 300 million tonnes)

of wheat which was suited to the dry steppes of the world. Besides the selection that occurs in nature, as illustrated by the example of wheat, man also intervenes by a deliberate process of selection, e.g. by his taste for glutinous or non-glutinous, long-grained or short-grained rice and so on. It is now possible to accelerate the processes of hybridisation and selection as well as to channel them in any desired direction, due to the growth in the science of plant genetics.

History has also intervened in several instances to bring about the spread of various crops. For example, potato was restricted to the Andean Highlands of South America until the sixteenth century when it was introduced to Europe. After a few decades of acclimatisation it emerged in a form suitable for the climatic conditions of Europe and eventually became a staple food. Sugar-cane was indigenous to Asia and was introduced all round the Mediterranean by the Arabs in the ninth century. Christopher Columbus took specimens with him on his second voyage to the Antilles in 1493, and the following year it reached Hispaniola and Cuba. By the early sixteenth century it was widely consumed, with sugar refineries established in Europe and a lucrative trade across the Atlantic. Cottonseed as a major source of edible oil is a development of this century and it is now widely used as a 'filler' oil in many powdered milks for infant feeding.

The dominance of a crop in any particular region is a result of a number of ecological factors. The soil, the environmental temperature, rainfall and number of hours of sunlight will determine which crop will grow best. Sociocultural and economic factors also depend on these. The farmer tends to concentrate his labour on a proven low-risk crop and to minimise diversity, but this also has its problems, because the farmer and his family will be restricted to one predominant source of nutrients and run the risk of deficiencies.

SYSTEMS THROUGH WHICH MAN INTERACTS WITH ENVIRONMENT TO OBTAIN FOOD

As human society has evolved and the knowledge of agriculture and farming has increased, man has evolved increasingly complex systems through which land can be worked and food obtained and processed for use. At one end of the spectrum is the traditional farming system, characteristic of the peasant societies of the Third World. Such a system involves only man, his animals, his seed and his land, with very little involvement of industry, government or commercial and other agencies. In such a system productivity of the land is limited by the fertility of the soil and the climate, and family income largely depends on the amount of land that can be worked with family labour. Three-quarters of the world's population still depend upon the products of their own field and agricultural labour to feed and provide for themselves. At the other end of the spectrum is the mechanised farm which forms part of the 'agribusiness', producing large crop surpluses. To compare outputs in the two systems, the average Indian or Pakistani farmer harvests little more than 1 tonne of rice or wheat per hectare against 6 tonnes in the USA. On the other hand, the latter uses up a disproportionate amount of energy to produce food calories. For example, in traditional societies 5-50 food calories are obtained for each calorie of energy invested. Industrialised societies require 5-10 calories of fuel energy to obtain 1 food calorie. Some modern wheat-growers can manage only 2.2 calories, sugar beet 0.49 calories and broiler chicken 0.11 calories for every calorie expended. Modernised agriculture may make economic sense but is not 'cost-efficient' where energy input and returns are concerned.

Agricultural technology

Many of the farming systems of the developing world use a minimum of technology. Human muscle or draught animals provide the force for working the land. External inputs in the forms of machines, fuels, pesticides and fertilisers are minimal or non-existent. The fertility of the soil is a limiting factor in output, particularly with regard to the nitrogen content, in which tropical soils tend to be deficient. The local varieties of grain grown are particularly suited to the environment, having been bred over a period of thousands of years, though the output is low. The traditional systems represent a type of ecological equilibrium which can be sustained indefinitely, given the available resources and provided that population growth is kept within the capacity of the system. On the other hand, modernisation in agriculture needs heavy inputs in the form of energy, fertilisers, irrigation and high maintenance as well as research costs.

Much of agriculture in the Third World is rain-dependent. In a system where, because of low production, the margin of safety is low, a deficiency of even 25 per cent in rainfall can lead to crop failure of sufficient intensity to give rise to a threat of famine. In many parts of Asia and Africa such a deficiency in rainfall occurs on average once in 5 years.

Extension programmes specifically developed to help the small landholders, and involving minimal capital expenditure, are necessary to improve agricultural outputs in the developing world. The 'gardening' system of agriculture, like intercropping (more than one crop in the field), multiple cropping (several crops in succession in a year), relay planting (sowing a second crop between the rows of an earlier maturing crop), together with composting and irrigation through wells, needs to be developed in order to improve food production in regions which suffer from chronic hunger. How much increase in productivity can be achieved by simple improvements can be appreciated by following the agricultural history of many of the more developed nations. For example, ratios of seed grown to grain harvested in medieval England, were of the order of 5 to 6 for wheat. In the eighteenth century, up-and-down husbandry (alternation of grass and tillage) increased yields for wheat and barley some 20-fold.

Social systems

Besides agricultural technology, social systems determine the amount of food available to an individual and his family. Inadequate nutrition has often been described as a *social* disease and in countries where malnutrition is common, its causes include factors inherent in the very nature of the society. Similarly, in countries where malnutrition has been overcome rapidly, political improvements have been major contributory factors.

In the typical developing country 50-80 per cent of the population is rural. The source of livelihood is the production of food or fibre crops or animal husbandry. The productivity of land is abysmally low; furthermore the ratio of land to population is dwindling. Thus in India the average size of a holding is 3.2 ha, but about 70 per cent of all holdings are below this average. Twenty-two per cent of rural families own no land at all and 47 per cent own less than 0.4 ha. In Bangladesh the number of landless families has currently reached more than 3 million. This increase of landless at a rate of 5 per cent a year and up to 20 per cent in some regions during 1972-74 cannot be explained by demographic reasons only. It is the small farmer, together with the growing number of the landless and the unemployed, who lack the soil, the water, the fertiliser as well as the economic and political power to feed themselves. The land tenure system in many countries favours the big landlord who employs farm labour at low wages. These are the farmers who tend to be favoured by governments' policies of restricting agricultural projects and grants to those with lands large enough to produce marketable surplus. In one study of rural poverty in India it was found that 40 per cent of the rural population had an annual per capita consumer expenditure below the estimated breadline.

The rural poor have limited access to health care and education. Housing is substandard and life-expectancy is low. Many are tied to a life of drudgery, eking out an existence on meagre land resources. In many such traditional agricultural systems almost half the energy derived by people and animals from the photosynthetic product of plants is expended to grow and prepare food, leaving little margin for anything else.

At the international level the social system also tends to favour the rich. Many countries in Africa and Asia are former colonies in which the best land was principally utilised for the production of cash crops. Fifty-five per cent of crop land in the Philippines, and over 80 per cent in Mauritius, is assigned to cash crops. In Cuba at one time huge areas of land were used for planting sugar and the production of food crops was in inverse proportion to the effort put into sugar production. In one of the provinces of the Dominican Republic three-quarters of arable land is controlled by a sugar producer, and the acreage under sugar has doubled in the last 20 years. Moreover, the thrust of agricultural research was also towards cash crops and local food crops were neglected. There are numerous centres for research on coffee, cocoa, oil palm, jute, rubber and cotton, but few for wheat, rice, maize and legumes. In more recent times the inequality of the international social system has taken yet another turn. The rising affluence of the industrialised nations has brought about a change in eating habits, causing an increased demand for meat and dairy products. This in turn has led to an increased demand for grain as cattle feed. In North America the per capita consumption of grain is about 1000 kg per year; of this, only about 75 kg are used directly as human food, much of the remainder being fed to animals. By contrast, cereal consumption in the Third World is about 200 kg per year, most of it being used as human food. Thus, the richer third of the world consumes half the available cereals. Three-quarters of the grain trade of the USA is with well-fed Europe, as are over half of the exports of soya bean. As a result cereal prices have risen faster than prices of cash crops like tea, cocoa, palm oil and sugar. It is estimated that net imports of 85 million tonnes of cereals will be needed in the Third World if agricultural output does not rise rapidly. Thus, food grain is likely to become a major political lever in the coming decades. Already in many of the food-exporting countries the farming lobby wields strong political influence.

Cultural factors

Agriculture has evolved with man and his culture. Since growing food is the main productive activity of rural areas, the agricultural systems used are very much part of the culture of a people. Thus there are several cultures in which cattle, and especially the bull, are given great importance. Land and its productivity are important in many peasant societies of tropical Africa. The festivities and carnivals in all rural societies are related to farming activities, e.g. spring festivals (to invoke fertility) and late summer harvest festivals (for thanksgiving and rejoicing).

Cultural practices also determine how the land will be worked. For example, in some parts of Africa which grow cash crops, men work the plot of land set aside for the cash crop and women work on a separate family plot to grow food. The *type* of work may also be divided according to sex. Men hoe (or plough) the land and sow, while women do the weeding and harvesting.

Religion and culture often determine the choice of foods. Many communities classify foods as 'hot' and 'cold' and avoid food combinations that are thought to be deleterious. The caste system in India determines not only the types of food that an individual may eat or abstain from, but also the person who may cook the food, the person(s) with whom he may take food and the rituals to be followed at meals.

In addition to the 'hot' and 'cold' classification there are 'light' foods to be eaten during illnesses, there are celebration foods for specific festivals (e.g. the Christmas turkey in the West; the Onam festival of Kerala, India, which is celebrated with 22 varieties of preparations from root vegetables), there are foods which people abstain from on certain days (e.g. meat on Fridays) and there are foods for entertaining important visitors.

From the nutritional point of view, cultural practices are more important in the case of certain vulnerable groups. In most societies food taboos and practices are directed at the pregnant woman and her child. In many cultures the pregnant woman is advised to eat less so that she will have an easy labour. Lamb meat and eggs are not allowed throughout pregnancy because of their supposed effects on the fetus. Similarly, there are several weaning practices which are harmful to the infant, e.g. abrupt weaning by separating the infant from the mother, the type of food introduced, the form and composition of the weaning foods offered, etc.

The various beliefs and dietary practices of a community are one of the many predisposing factors in malnutrition. An important *precipitating* factor in most instances is infection. The nutritional needs of the body are increased during an episode of illness, when the appetite is often decreased: in addition, various foods are withheld in the mistaken belief that such a practice hastens recovery. The practice of 'starving a cold' is well known. Similarly, food is often withheld from a child suffering from diarrhoea, measles and other febrile illnesses. The effect of bad dietary practices is greatest during bouts of illness, when the nutritional status of the individual deteriorates rapidly.

The common cultural patterns and beliefs related to foods are summarised in Table 1.1.

Table 1.1 *Prevailing cultural patterns and beliefs related to food in different regions*

South America[1]
Classification of foods into 'hot' and 'cold' widely practised in South America and dates back to the Spanish influences since the sixteenth century. There is a great deal of variation in the classification between individual countries.

Hot	Cold
Cereals, sugar, some meats, alcohol, edible oil, pumpkins.	Fruits, vegetables, milk and pork

Bread is considered templado or temperate. Hot foods are generally preferred and considered better for health e.g. in coastal Peru beef (hot) is preferred over fish or mutton (cold).

Central America[2]
'Hot' and 'cold' classification is widespread but becoming less strong on account of exposure to modern concepts and emergence of 'fresco' or neutral foods.

Hot	Cold
Cereal grains, chillies, most temperate zone fruits, goat's milk, high-prestige meats (like beef, mutton, waterfowl) most edible oils and aromatic beverages.	Maize, fresh vegetables, beans, squash, most tropical fruits, dairy products, low-prestige meats like goat, fish and chicken.

Caribbean[3]
'Hot' and 'cold' beliefs are prevalent, but are also being influenced by taste and flavour preferences. Appearance is also a factor in food selection, e.g. white polished rice preferred to grey par-boiled kind. Imported foods and particularly imported canned foods have a prestige value.
Common 'hot' foods are milk, eggs and maize. Melon, pineapple, coconut-water mango and soursop are considered cold foods.

South Africa[3,4]
No 'hot', 'cold' classification but various food taboos. Fish is generally disliked. Generally food restrictions favour men over women, e.g. eggs, game meat, etc. Class or totemic taboos are prevalent.
Imported foods like refined cereals, carbonated drinks and sweets often have high prestige value.

East Africa[5]
Fish, eggs, fowl generally considered distasteful, unclean or liable to cause sterility or thievery. Food restrictions, especially of protein-rich foods, favour men. Eggs, chicken and mutton are generally restricted foods for all women with additional restrictions in pregnancy.

West Africa[6]

Some foods, usually the local staples, are believed to have mystical properties and are considered 'superfoods'.

Egg taboo is widely prevalent. Meat, poultry and fish are often given sparingly to women and children.

Seasonal agricultural cycle has resulted in festivals and religious feasts.

North Africa and the Near East[7,8]

Food has a semi-religious status. Wasting food is a 'sin'. The kitchen or cooking areas are holy, and quarrels, abusive language or entry of strangers are not allowed. Sharing of food is the common practice.

Many food taboos exist and apply especially to children.

Bread has a special status and is referred to as 'the staff of life'.

Pork is avoided, as are also certain types of meat and fish.

Fasting during the month of Ramadhan common in all Moslem communities.

East and South-east Asia[9,10]

Rice is often synonymous to 'food', partly because of its bulk and filling capacity. Polished white rice is considered prestige food.

Indigenous medical practices attribute various qualities to different foods, and prescribe special diets for illness.

'Hot' and 'cold' classification common in Burma, Malaysia, Philippines and Indonesia.

Pork is avoided in Muslim countries.

Central Asia[11,12]

The Hindu, Ayurvedic and Muslim 'Unani' systems of indigenous medicine classify foods as 'hot' and 'cold' based on their supposedly heating and cooling effects on the body. Illness and various physiological states like menstruation or pregnancy are classified as being 'hot' or 'cold'. An individual in a 'hot' state must avoid eating 'hot' foods and instead consume more 'cold' foods to help neutralise the condition.

Hot foods	Cold foods
Most animal proteins such as meats, poultry, eggs, fish, refined butter (ghee), some vegetable proteins and buffalo milk. Cereals like wheat or sorghum and some vegetable oils like mustard oil are believed to be 'hot'. Papaya, mango, jackfruit, cabbage, cauliflower and sweet potato are amongst the vegetables considered 'hot'. Honey, jaggery, tea, coffee and most spices are considered 'hot'.	Milk of goat and cow as well as dairy products like yogurt, buttermilk and milk curds. Most legumes and pulses are thought to be 'cold'. Fruits and vegetables generally are considered 'cooling', especially cucumbers, citrus fruit and green leafy vegetables.

Within the 'hot'/'cold' classification there are other systems of grouping foods, e.g. 'gassy' foods which are avoided during stomach upsets.

Introduction

The concept of 'sanctity of life' in Hinduism contributes to a predominantly lacto-vegetarian diet, and pork as well as various types of fish are avoided by Moslems.

Fasting is a common practice amongst the Hindu, and fasting during the month of Ramadhan obligatory for all Moslems.

1. Mintz, A. M. J. and Vanveen, A. G. A sociological approach to a dietary survey and food habits study in an Andean community. *Trop. Geog. Med.* (1968), **20**, 88.
2. Cosminsky, S. Alimento and Fresco – nutritional concepts and their implications for health care. *Hum. Org.* (1977), **36** (2), 203.
3. Moore, F. W. Food habits in non-industrial societies. In Dupon, J. (ed.) *Dimensions of Nutrition: Proceedings.* Colorado Associated University Press, 1970.
4. McLellan, D. L. and May, J. *The Ecology of Malnutrition in Seven Countries of South Africa and in Portuguese Guinea.* Hafner Press, N.Y., 1971.
5. Campbell, R. M. and Cuthbertson, D. P. Factors influencing man's selection of food. In Cuthbertson, D. P. (ed.) *Progress in Nutrition and Allied Sciences.* Boyd, Edinburgh, 1963.
6. Osuntokun, B. O. Nutrition problems in the African region. *Bull. Schweiz Med. Wiss.* (1976), **31**, 353.
7. Todhunter, E. Neige. Food habits, for faddism and nutrition. *World Rev. Nutr. Diet.* (1973), **16**, 286.
8. Patwardhan, V. N. *et al. The State of Nutrition in the Arab Middle East.* Vanderbilt University Press, Nashville, Tenn., 1972.
9. Tan Mely, G. *Social and Cultural Aspects of Food Patterns and Food Habits in Five Rural Areas in Indonesia.* National Institute of Economic and Social Research and Directorate of Nutrition Dept. of Health, Republic of Indonesia, Jakarta, 1970.
10. Guthrie, H. A. Infant feeding practices in 5 communities groups in the Philippines. *J. Trop. Ped.* (1964), **10**, 65.
11. Amin, A. and Zeitlin, M. *Index of Unani and Traditional Food Values of Pakistani Foods.* U.S.A.I.D. July 1972.
12. Athavale, V. B. Bala-veda. *Ped. Clin. India,* 1977.

Storage and utilisation of food

The crop which is harvested is stored and processed before it is cooked and eaten. During each of these steps nutrients may be altered or lost. For example, if storage facilities are inadequate, much of the foodgrain may be lost to insects and rodents. In some cases the losses may amount to almost a third of the total crop. Food can also deteriorate during storage because of fungal growth caused by temperature and humidity and lack of aeration. Thus aflatoxin can affect both ground nuts and other food crops, resulting in health hazards to the consumers. India alone has an estimated annual loss of food in storage equal to the sum of food aid for the entire world. In France a third of all bread produced is discarded for one reason or another. In the United States a Congressional report found that in 1974 the equivalent of 24 million hectares of farmland and 9 million tonnes of fertiliser were used to produce food that was not consumed. More recent research indicates that grain storage at the level of the village home or the small farm is important, and improvements in the traditional ways of storing grain are urgently needed. In many countries village craftsmen can be utilised to produce improved receptacles for storage or village silos.

Apart from vegetables and fruits, most food crops are processed before eating. The aim of such processing is to reduce bulk, improve digestibility, improve appearance, add flavours and increase palatability. Many methods of processing also help the keeping qualities of the crop, so that it can be stored for a prolonged period of time.

The commonest form of processing is milling, either for altering flavour or for polishing, as in the case of rice. In the case of both, the outer layers of the grain are discarded as bran. All nutrients are not evenly distributed in the grain. For example, the two outer layers

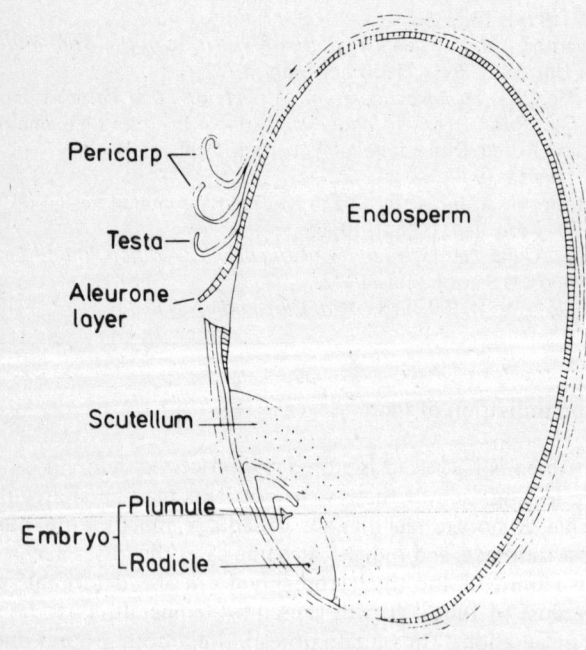

Figure 1.6   Longitudinal section of cereal grain

(aleurone and scutellum (figure 1.6)) comprise 8.5 per cent of the weight of the grain and contain 94 per cent of thiamine, 51 per cent of riboflavin, 83 per cent of niacin and 21 per cent of the protein of the grain. The highly refined flour or polished rice can be made into attractive white bread or cooked white rice, but will be devoid of nutrients as well as fibre, and will consist principally of starch. In most rural societies home pounding or stone grinding, with or without prior fermenting, is the common method of preparing flour from the cereal, but the method is time-consuming and laborious and the flour is coarse and gritty, so that these practices are gradually being abandoned in favour of the village mill.

Parboiling of rice is a processing method used in some of the rural areas where rice is a staple food. It has been estimated that more than a sixth of the rice consumed is treated by parboiling. The grain is soaked, steamed and dried carefully. During the soaking, nutrients pass from the outer into the inner parts of the grain and the germ becomes more firmly attached during drying. Because of this, the grain loses fewer nutrients during milling. Also the outer coats become hardened and resistant to insects. The processing of food is considered further in Chapter 2.

Processing in the home and the kitchen

In addition to commercial or large-scale processing, food may be processed in the home before it is cooked. For example, in many areas where cassava is a staple, it must be soaked in water, pounded and washed several times to get rid of the cyanide toxins present in the tuber; however, nutrients are also lost in the process. Legumes and beans are germinated until they sprout before they are cooked. Vitamin C is synthesised during germination and the concentration of certain vitamins of the B group is also increased during sprouting.

Many foods are fermented before they are eaten. Soya beans and ground nuts are treated in this manner to produce pastes or cheese. The process helps to improve the digestibility of the food, and the vitamin content also increases.

Cooking may involve some loss of nutrients, e.g. when vegetables are boiled in water and then all excess water is drained off before serving. Similarly, excess washing of cereals, especially rice to make it look white instead of brown, will result in loss of nutrients, as shown in Table 1.2. During cooking various foods absorb water at different rates, producing different amounts of bulk. The caloric density, i.e. the number of calories per unit volume of food eaten, is important especially in children and other vulnerable groups in communities subsisting on

Table 1.2 Percentage loss of nutrients through washing

	Thiamine	Riboflavin	Nicotinic acid
Husked rice	21	8	13
Milled rice	20	26	23
Parboiled rice	15	15	13
Home pounded rice	7	12	10

Table 1.3 Effects of boiling potato and rice

	Percentage of water		Protein/100 g of cooked product	
	Raw	Boiled	Raw	Boiled
Potato	76	81	2.1	1.4
Rice	12	70.88	6.8	2.3-1.0

marginal nutrition. Thus both rice and potato absorb water in differing proportions so that the calories or protein per 100 g of cooked rice or creamed potato are very different from those in the raw foods.

The food industry

Rapid urbanisation and affluence have created a demand for pre-cooked and convenience foods, with supermarket chains and a variety of industry and business interests providing the supply of such foods. This 'agribusiness' has spawned giant multinationals with business interests extending from farm machinery and fertilisers to packaging and shipping of the finished products. In the 'granary' countries of the industrial world the multinationals have increasingly come to control the growing and procuring of food. They can thus influence world supplies as well as prices of essential foods. In many cases there is over-enthusiastic promotion of the packaged foods, which influences eating habits even in well-informed societies. Between 1959 and 1970 the consumption of fruit and vegetables declined in the USA by more than a fifth. Consumption of milk dropped 20 per cent, while that of soft drinks went up 79 per cent. The sales of potato crisps went up 85 per cent, and ice cream 29 per cent. Processed convenience food does not necessarily give the customer the best value for money. For example, corn costing US$2.95 a bushel, when processed into Cocoa Puffs (corn meal, sugar, corn syrup, cocoa, salt, etc.) fetches $75 a bushel, and puffed wheat under the name of Quaker Oats fetches $110 per bushel. There is also the added hint that such products have captured the 'goodness of sunshine' and are health-promoting! The effects of such promotion are seen at their maximum in rural areas of the developing countries where white bread, cola drinks and biscuits have become prestige items and scant family resources are being spent on food items with little nutritive value.

This brief outline of the social, cultural, technical and commercial factors in the production and utilisation of food provides a background against which nutritional deficiencies occur in individuals, families and communities. In their turn nutritional deficiencies affect the health of the people concerned. The following pages describe the prevalence of individual nutritional disorders, their relationship to health, and discuss methods of prevention.

FURTHER READING

Dumont, R. and Cohen, N. *The Growth of Hunger. A new politics of agriculture.* Marion Boyars, London and Boston, 1980.
George, S. *How the Other Half Dies. The real reasons for world hunger.* Penguin Books, Middlesex, 1976.
Lappe, F. M., Collins, J. and Fowler, C. *Food First : beyond the myth of scarcity.* Houghton Mifflin Co., Boston, 1977.
Tudge, C. *The Famine Business.* Penguin Books, Middlesex, 1977.

Chapter 2

Common Tropical Foods

Man's domestication of plants to produce adequate and dependable supplies of food enabled the transition from the hunter-gatherer stage to living in settled communities. Many would regard this as a major leap forward in the civilisation of man since it marked the beginnings of development along several fronts including social, political and economic sciences as well as in agricultural and food sciences. Cereals were the first plants to be domesticated from amongst the various grass plants. Each of the world's great civilisations has depended upon cereal as a food source. The earliest actual remains of grain date from around 5000 BC. It seems that the basic crop of Neolithic agriculture in the fertile crescent was a primitive form of wheat – einkorn and wild emmer wheat. This continued until the Bronze Age when the production of emmer and einkorn decreased and barley became more popular. The cultivation of rice has been traced as far back as 3000 BC. Today cereals represent the world's most important source of food, and failure of cereal crop anywhere in the world will threaten to bring malnutrition and starvation to millions.

All cereals are seeds of plants which evolved from the grasses. All of them contain the starchy endosperm as the main part. For example, in the case of wheat, the endosperm constitutes 80-85 per cent of the seed. It is separated from the testa by a proteinous layer called the aleurone layer. The embryo, forming only about 3 per cent of the seed, is situated at the base of the seed. The scutellum lies between the endosperm and the embryo. During germination the scutellum secretes enzymes which digest the endosperm and transfer the digested food substances to the growing part of the embryo. Thus the scutellum carries out the triple function of digesting, absorbing and transferring food to the embryo.

The importance of cereals in the dietaries of developing countries is much greater than in the case of affluent societies. For example, in many countries of Western Europe and North America the staple cereal wheat provides less than 30 per cent of total calories in the average diet.

Even amongst some relatively poor communities, the contribution to total calories from wheat and wheat products rarely exceeds 60 per cent. By contrast, in most developing countries up to 70 per cent of total calories are derived from the staple cereals like rice, maize or sorghum. Hence the form in which the cereals are consumed is important. Losses of nutrients in processing can easily lead to deficiency disorders since these nutrients cannot be adequately supplied from the small amounts of other accompanying foods. Secondly, all food crops in the developing world are grown on small farms using simple technologies which are highly labour-intensive. For example, more than 100 million farms in the developing world are smaller than 5 ha, and 50 million are less than 1 ha. Less than 20 per cent of the farmers in the developing world have access to fertilisers. Furthermore, small farmers are unable to store their products or pace their harvests to suit their nutritional needs. They tend to suffer low prices for their produce at harvest times and later high prices as consumers during the hungry months. Food losses on the field and during storage, from rodents and insects, can be considerable. For example, in 1965 the United States spent US$3 billion on pest-control. By contrast, the peasant farmer in the developing world can spend very little to protect his crop. It is therefore not surprising that even though food production in the developing world has increased over the decades, it has not been able to keep pace with population growth, with the result that many countries have now to depend on imports of cereals to feed their populations. Food has now become an important factor in international trade as well as a powerful political weapon.

THE MAJOR CEREALS

Wheat

Wheat is of great importance: in agriculture with a total world production above 400 million tonnes; in trade with more than a fifth of the world's wheat crop being for export; and in nutrition with more than 1000 million people being dependent on it. The last 150 years have seen an enormous increase in the world production of wheat. General improvements in agricultural techniques in the Western world have been largely related to growing wheat with high efficiency. New varieties of wheat have been evolved by plant scientists, chiefly with the object of increasing yield and of raising resistance to disease.

There are three principle varieties: *Triticum vulgare*, *T. durum* and *T. compactum*. *T. vulgare* is the principal variety used for breadmaking, for cakes and biscuits. *T. durum* is used for semolina products. Spring wheat and winter wheat are different in the characteristics of their flour on account of differences in protein content. Gluten is the main protein of wheat. During breadmaking the gas produced by fermentation stretches the gluten in which bubbles of gas are trapped giving rise to porous bread. In general, flours of high gluten content make better bread.

Breadmaking in the world as a whole ranges between two extremes. At one end, as in most peasant societies, bread is made at home by roasting, baking or frying unfermented dough and is unleavened, e.g. chapatis. At the other end is the factory loaf made from standardised flour and after a period of fermentation and baking.

Wheat is usually ground into flour and very rarely used as the whole cereal. The nutritional value of the flour depends upon the degree of milling or, as it is commonly called, the extraction rate. In most peasant communities *stone milling* is common. This process crushes or grinds the entire grain, and the more fibrous parts of the grain which are not reduced to powder get sieved as bran. The germ and scutellum which are oily tend to get pressed into flat particles and may get sieved off. However, the modern method of *roller-milling* has now become more common and all larger national milling corporations use this new technology. Here the processing of grinding occurs in two stages. In the first stage corrugated rollers break off parts of the grain and the reduced grain is then ground in the second stage by smooth rollers. In this process it is possible to have the flour coming out in streams, and by adjusting the streams the miller can control the extraction rate. In many Western countries the common wheat flour is of between 70 and 72 per cent extraction rate. The flour is then enriched by the addition of calcium (as chalk), iron and vitamins, including vitamin C. For example, in the UK the law demands that each 100 g flour should contain 0.24 mg thiamine, 1.6 mg nicotinic acid, 1.65 mg iron, and calcium carbonate in amounts not less than 235 mg and not in excess of 390 mg. The lower the extraction rate of the flour, the whiter it is in appearance, and the better are its keeping qualities. But loss of nutrients is also greater. Table 2.1 gives the composition of flour at different rates of extraction.

In the grain trade the different varieties of wheat are commonly spoken of as 'durum', 'hard' or 'soft'. These terms reflect the characteristics of the milled product; whether it is hard and granular or soft and fluffy. Durum wheat is used to make spaghetti, macaroni and other pastas. Hard wheat has a higher protein content and is superior for breadmaking, and soft wheat is preferred for cakes, biscuits and so on.

In different countries the bakers may add various substances to

Table 2.1 Composition of wheat flour (per 100 g) at different extraction rates

	72% extraction	80% extraction	95-100% (wholemeal)
Water (g)	14.5	14	14
kcalories	337	327	318
Protein (g)	11.3	12.8	13.2
Iron (mg)	2.2[a]	3.6[a]	
	1.5[b]	2.5[b]	4.0
Calcium	140[a]	150[a]	
	15[b]	20[b]	35
Thiamine (mg)	0.31[a]	0.42[a]	
	0.10[b]	0.30[b]	0.46
Niacin (mg)	2.0[a]	4.2[a]	
	0.7[b]	1.7[b]	5.6
Riboflavin (mg)	0.035	0.05	0.08
Pantothenic acid (mg)	0.6	0.9	1.5
Pyridoxine (mg)	0.15	0.25	0.5
Biotin (mg)	—	—	0.007

[a] Fortified flour.
[b] Unfortified flour.

wheat flour in breadmaking. For example, skimmed milk powder may be added to the extent of 5-6 per cent in many countries. In Egypt yoghourt is mixed with dough. Soya flour to the extent of 2 per cent, and sugar, are added in several countries of South America. In developing countries cassava flour may be added, sometimes up to 30 per cent, for economic reasons. On the other hand soya or ground nut flour may be added to improve the nutrient content of bread. The nutrient contents of bread and chapati are compared in table 2.2.

Bulgar wheat is being increasingly provided by various donor agencies. It is parboiled wheat prepared either by steaming or by boiling wheat grain with a small quantity of water until all the water is absorbed. The keeping qualities of wheat are improved by this process. It can be prepared for eating by steaming or boiling. A little oil or stock is then added to the cooked product for taste.

Table 2.2 *Nutrient contents of bread and chapati (per 100 g)*

	Water (g)	Kcal.	Protein (g)	Fat (g)	Carbo-hydrates (g)	Calcium (mg)	Iron (mg)	Thiamine (mg)	Nicotinic acid (mg)
Wholemeal bread	40.0	216	8.8	2.7	41.8	23	2.5	0.26	3.9
Brown bread	39.0	223	8.9	2.2	44.7	100	2.5	0.24	2.9
White bread	39.0	233	7.8	1.7	49.7	100	1.7	0.18	1.4
Chapati made with fat	28.5	336	8.1	12.8	50.2	66	2.3	0.26	1.7
Chapati with no fat	45.8	202	7.3	1.0	43.7	60	2.1	0.23	1.5

Rice

Rice is the staple food for more than half of mankind. No wonder that ancient Sanskrit literature described rice as 'the sustainer of the human race'. The present world production of rice amounts to nearly 400 million tonnes, almost 90 per cent of it being grown in Asia, although some rice is also grown in Europe, North and South America, and Australia. Unlike wheat, most of the world's crop of rice is produced on smallholdings by labour-intensive methods. It is estimated that over 1000 man-hours per hectare are required for the cultivation of rice. Most rice is grown under water and the fields need to be under water to a depth of several centimetres during the greater part of the growing season. These requirements reflect the origins of rice as a swamp plant. New varieties are being developed for growing on different terrains and for high yield.

About 74 per cent of the paddy is available as rice or its by-products. The nutrient content of rice is influenced by the variety, the condition of the soil and the application of fertilisers. However, the most important effect on nutrient content is that of processing prior to use. The structure of the rice grain is such that the outer layers can be easily removed by simple mechanical means such as, for example, milling. During the last half-century or so mechanical milling has replaced the practice of home pounding. During milling the pericarp, aleurone layer and the germ are removed. Protein, fat, vitamins and minerals occur in greater amounts in the germ and the outer layers compared to the starchy endosperm. Losses of nutrients due to milling have been found to be 76 per cent for thiamine, 56 per cent for riboflavin and 63 per cent for niacin. Up to 17 per cent of protein may be lost on account of milling. Another effect of milling is that the removal of the outer protective seed coats facilitates the extraction of soluble substances during washing of rice prior to cooking as described in table 1.2 on page 14. Table 2.3 gives further details of the losses in individual nutrients.

Table 2.3 Losses of nutrients during washing of rice (nutrient contents expressed as µg/g)

	Thiamine			Riboflavin			Niacin		
	Before	After	Loss(%)	Before	After	Loss(%)	Before	After	Loss(%)
Husked	4.40	3.47	21.14	0.65	0.60	7.70	54.00	47.00	13.00
Milled	0.65	0.37	43.07	0.27	0.20	25.92	20.57	15.83	23.04
Undermilled	2.94	2.75	6.46	0.38	0.34	10.52	50.00	42.00	16.00
Parboiled	3.02	2.82	6.62	0.41	0.36	12.19	49.00	44.00	10.20

Source: Kik, M. C. and Williams, R. R. *Bulletin 112*, National Research Council (USA), Washington, 1945

In the past, milling also included polishing. Special polishing powders were used to give a white glossy appearance to the grain. This unnecessary and objectionable practice is now being given up, particularly because some of the polishing powders used by the millers have been found to be harmful. Several countries now demand a standard content of nutrients by law. For example, the US standard requires that 1 lb (450 g) of rice must contain 2-4 mg thiamine, 1.2-2.4 mg riboflavin, 16-32 mg niacin and 13-26 mg iron.

In several countries, for example India, paddy is treated by parboiling as described on page 13. Rice is soaked for 1 or 2 days, after which it is steamed for 30 minutes or less and then dried in the sun. During the process the various water-soluble nutrients, which are largely concentrated in the germ and the aleurone layer, diffuse into the grain. When these parts of the grain are removed during milling, the loss of nutrients is not excessive. Up to 20 per cent of the rice crop in India is treated in this traditional manner, which also improves the keeping qualities of rice.

Most rice is consumed boiled, with a sufficient amount of water for all of it to be absorbed. If excess water is used and then some discarded towards the end, a considerable loss of nutrients can occur. All excess water should be recycled either as stock or for cooking vegetables. During cooking the grain absorbs a considerable amount of water and the nutritional value of boiled rice is a great deal different from that of the raw grain (table 2.4).

Table 2.4 Nutritional value of raw and boiled rice (per 100 g)

	Water (g)	kcal.	Protein (g)	Fat (g)	Carbo-hydrates (g)	Calcium (mg)	Iron (mg)	Thiamine (mg)	Ribo-flavin (mg)	Niacin (mg)
Raw rice (milled)	11.7	361	6.5	1.0	86.8	4	0.5	0.08	0.03	1.5
Boiled rice	69.9	123	2.2	0.3	29.6	1	0.2	0.01	0.01	0.3

Maize

Maize originated in the New World and was introduced into Europe at the end of the fifteenth century. It was the main staple of the Incas, Mayas and the Aztecs, together with potato. It is widely grown in America extending from the Platta valley to the Mississippi valley. Maize is also the main staple of many communities in Africa. The world production of maize is about 250 million tonnes.

The way maize has spread globally from its origin in America indicates its remarkable adaptability. Unlike wheat and rice, which are limited by climatic conditions, maize flourishes in a variety of different soils, latitudes, altitudes and weather conditions. Maize provides a high yield of food energy at a relatively lower expense of seed and labour (table 2.5). It is also a sturdy plant and is protected against damage by birds and insects.

Table 2.5 Yields (tonne/ha) of different cereals and other staple foods

	Wheat	Rice (milled)	Maize	Sweet potato	Cassava
Average yield	1.08	0.914	1.6	4.596	4.596
Calories (million/ha)	3.22	4.16	5.36	4.509	5.567

The maize kernel, like that of other cereal grains, includes the inner endosperm, the germ and the outer layers which constitute the bran. The endosperm makes up 80 per cent of the grain and contains over 80 per cent of the starch and 75 per cent of the protein. The aleurone layer contains 20 per cent of the protein. The germ, constituting 10 per cent of the grain, contains all the oil and most of the minerals. The nutrient content varies according to the strain. For example, the protein content can vary from 15 to 6 per cent. Maize is the richest amongst cereals in fat content and some strains may contain up to 7 per cent of fat in the grain though the average is 4.5 per cent. Maize oil is a good source of linoleic and oleic acids.

The principal protein of maize is zein which constitutes half the total protein. On hydrolysis zein yields very little tryptophan and lysine. Recent research has led to the production of new strains of maize with high lysine content. Opaque-2 and Floury-2 have much less zein but high amounts of lysine; in some varieties tryptophan content is as high as 50 per cent.

The vitamins are mainly located in the germ and the outermost layers of endosperm, including the aleurone. This distribution is the same as in other cereals and is important from the milling point of view.

Maize has three major uses: as a staple food for many parts of the world, feed for livestock, and in industry. Much of the maize used for human consumption is not industrially processed, and the more nutritious parts of the grain are retained. Maize has thus an advantage over wheat and rice. Home processing may also help to add nutrients to the grain. For example, in parts of Latin America the whole grains are subjected to alkali treatment by soaking in lime water before grinding into flour. This helps to raise the calcium content of the flour.

Modern technology of milling is now catching up, especially in urban areas. During milling the kernel is gradually reduced in such a way that large particles of the hull and the germ remain intact and are easily separated. 'Decorticated' maize meal has a substantial part of the outer fibrous layers of the kernel removed, so that the fibre content is reduced by a third. The bran layer contains a large proportion of minerals and these are lost. If portions of aleurone layer are also removed there is a further loss of nutrients. 'Degerminated' maize meal has both bran and the germ removed, and the loss of nutrients is that much more. The milling of maize into flour has economic advantages. The separation of bran and germ improves the keeping qualities of the flour. There are also various by-products of the milling process such as, for example, maize oil. Maize germ and maize germ meal are also of value in the feeding of livestock.

Maize is largely eaten as thin (fluid) or stiff porridge or in the form of flat unleavened bread roasted on an open fire. The nutritional quality of the diet will depend on the processing of the grain prior to cooking and also the accompaniments.

Sorghum

Sorghum is grown in the USA, Pakistan, Central India, Africa and China. The annual production of sorghum is in the region of 44 million tonnes. The main protein of sorghum is kafirin. The germ has a high fat content like maize and oil can be extracted from it. The major fatty acids of the oil from the germ of sorghum are palmitic, stearic, oleic and linoleic.

Sorghum and millet are adapted to a wide range of climatic conditions and yields are generally good in conditions unfavourable to most other cereals. In many countries average yields vary between 500 and 1700 kg per hectare, though the newer high-yield varieties give higher yields.

Sorghum and millet are mainly consumed in the form of thin or stiff porridge in most of Africa. In India, the flour is used to prepare flat unleavened bread roasted on fire. In the West, sorghum, like maize, is mainly used for the feeding of livestock.

TUBERS AND FRUITS USED AS STAPLE FOODS

Cassava

Cassava is grown in Indonesia, Malaysia, the Philippines, Thailand and parts of Africa and South America. In several communities it is the staple food. The plant is easily cultivated and is immune to most food pests. The major part of the plant used for food is the root although the leaves are also used as vegetables. There are two main varieties: the bitter cassava (*Manihot esculenta*) and the sweet cassava (*M. dulcis*). The bitter taste is due to large quantities of cyanide containing glycosides which must be removed by repeated washing of pounded cassava. This also removes most nutrients, leaving mainly starch behind. Cassava and other tubers contain very small amounts of protein, and can cause protein deficiency if eaten alone as the main foods.

The increasing popularity of cassava is a cause of concern. On account of ease of planting and growing, cassava is becoming the preferred crop for families where the head of the household works in the city and returns for brief periods to work on the family plot. The presence of cyanide in some varieties of cassava has been associated with the occurrence of tropical neuropathies where cassava is the main staple.

Plantains

Plantains are eaten as the main staple in several communities, especially in Africa. The high carbohydrate (20 per cent) and low protein (1 per cent) content of plantains is largely responsible for malnutrition in children weaned on a diet consisting largely of this staple.

Potato

Potato was brought to Europe from America and has become rapidly established in the European cuisine. From there it has spread to many countries and is now very widely grown. In the tropical dietaries potatoes make only a small contribution, being largely eaten as part of the vegetable dish of the day. As in other starchy tubers, the protein content of potato is small, being less than 2 per cent, but the protein is of good quality and is more easily available.

LEGUMES

Legumes are the edible seeds of plants which belong to the botanic family, Leguminosae. They play an important role both in tropical agriculture and in nutrition. The roots of many species have nodules which carry bacteria that are able to fix nitrogen. Thus, legumes tend to enrich the soil and are of great value in the rotation of crops. From the nutrition point of view, they have a larger protein content than most cereals and they are thus an important vegetable source of protein. The term 'poor man's meat' is all the more true since the amino acid sequence of most legumes is such that they complement the amino acids of cereal protein (table 2.6). Thus, a mixture of cereal and legumes

Table 2.6 *Amino acids in the proteins of common foods (g per 100 g protein)*

Amino acids	Wheat	Rice	Maize	Potato	Cassava	Ground nut	Average legume (e.g. beans)	Soya beans	Cow's milk	Eggs
Arginine	4.3	8.5	5.0	5.3	10.0	10.6	7.8	7.4	3.7	6.4
Valine	4.3	6.2	5.6	5.1	3.0	5.0	4.3	5.3	7.0	7.2
Histidine	2.1	2.2	2.4	1.4	1.5	2.4	3.1	2.6	2.7	2.6
Isoleucine	3.8	4.8	4.0	4.5	2.8	4.2	4.9	5.3	6.2	5.6
Leucine	6.4	8.2	12.0	4.6	4.1	6.2	7.7	7.7	9.9	9.0
Lysine	2.7	4.2	3.0	5.0	4.1	3.5	9.3	6.4	7.8	6.7
Methionine	1.6	2.1	2.1	1.6	0.6	1.0	0.9	1.3	2.4	3.0
Phenylalanine	4.6	4.6	5.0	4.2	2.8	5.0	4.6	5.0	5.1	5.3
Tyrosine	3.2	5.8	3.8	2.9	1.8	3.0	2.5	3.7	5.6	4.3
Threonine	2.9	3.5	4.2	3.7	2.8	2.9	5.9	4.0	4.6	5.3
Tryptophan	1.3	1.4	0.8	1.3	1.3	1.1	1.2	1.4	1.4	1.8

in the correct proportion can in theory provide all the amino acids needed by the body. Several legumes, like soya and ground nuts, are important sources of oil besides protein. They thus make a useful contribution to the diet by improving the nutrient density (i.e. quantity of nutrient per unit volume of food). Many legumes are eaten in the dried whole form without prior milling. Hence loss of nutrients because of the loss of outer layers, as in the milling of cereals, does not occur. Moreover, the commonest form of processing carried out in many homes is the prior sprouting of the legumes, e.g. sprout beans. During this process vitamin C is increased, the proportion of nicotinic acid is increased by between 50 and 100 per cent, and most starch is converted into sugar. It is well recognised that the constituents of the seed stored in an inert form begin to get organised in sprouting for supply to the embryo and may become more assimilable when eaten as food.

In the case of some legumes, toxic substances have been identified and these are of special importance. For example, in the case of the legume *Lathyrus sativus*, the presence of a toxic factor (B-oxalylamino acetic acid – BOAA) is responsible for causing paralysis. The disease, known as lathyrism, is crippling. A haemolytic factor is present in *Vicia faba* (fava beans) which can precipitate haemolytic anaemia in those with a deficiency of the enzyme glucose-6-phosphate dehydrogenase. In the case of ground nuts that have not been stored properly the growth of fungus can give rise to the presence of a toxic substance – aflatoxin.

The world production of legumes was estimated to be 48 million tonnes in 1980. A large proportion of world legume production consists of soya which is now increasingly produced outside Asia, chiefly in the United States. Even though soya production is being encouraged in countries with poor protein resources, it is unlikely that soya will become a part of the common diet except in the commercial powdered form. This is because, in Asia, soya is extensively processed prior to its use as food in order to improve taste and palatability as well as to destroy the anti-trypsin factor present in the bean. This type of kitchen technology, which is part of the tradition of one culture, is difficult to transfer to another culture.

EDIBLE OIL PLANTS

The fruits or seeds of several plants contain edible oil which can be expressed for human consumption or for industrial purposes. Many such plants are used as foods, e.g. maize or ground nuts, and are usually classified as cereals, vegetables, fruits or nuts. Since cooking oils and fats are relatively expensive there is very little frying in the everyday cooking of the peasant household in the developing world. The same is also true in the case of the urban poor. Except on festive occasions, most daily dishes are prepared by roasting, boiling or baking. On the other hand, energy deficiency has been identified as a major nutritional problem in the developing world. This is partly due to the bulkiness of the cereal staple and there is a need for improving the energy density of the traditional diet without of course increasing expense. One way of achieving this would be through identifying plants containing edible oil which can then be included in the daily food. Ground nuts and soya are two examples of this approach. Red palm oil is extensively used for everyday cooking in West Africa, and many coastal and island communities in the tropics use the coconut in a similar manner. Olive oil and sesame seeds or oil are common ingredients of diet in the Middle East, North Africa and other Mediterranean countries. Cotton seeds, sesame, sunflower seeds and rapeseeds are other common sources of oil.

MILK AND MILK PRODUCTS

It is estimated that about 65 per cent of the world's cattle are raised in the developing countries. But they provide only 20 per cent of the world's output of milk, and there is a need for improving milk output per head of cattle using modern knowledge. Amongst the pastoral communities milk is an important item of diet. Very little milk is drunk fresh, especially amongst the pastoral people of tropical Africa. A great deal of milk is soured and consumed as such. Yoghourt is popular in most of the Middle East, India and Pakistan. Cheese is not a common food as yet in most of the developing world. Like souring and yoghourt, cheesemaking will be another way of preventing spoilage and stretching the use of available milk. Table 2.7 gives the nutritional values of milk and some common milk products.

Table 2.7 *Nutrient content of milk and milk products (per 100 g)*

	Water (g)	kcal.	Protein (g)	Fat (g)	Carbo-hydrate (g)	Lactose (g)	Calcium (mg)	Iron (mg)
Cow's milk	87.6	65	3.3	3.8	4.7	4.7	120	0.05
Goat's milk	87.0	71	3.3	4.5	4.6	4.6	130	0.04
Yoghourt (low-fat cow's milk)	85.7	52	5.0	1.0	6.2	4.6	180	0.09
Cottage cheese	78.8	96	13.6	0.4	1.4	1.4	60	0.10
Chedder-type cheese	37.0	406	26.0	33.5	Tr.	Tr.	800	0.40

PREPARING A BALANCED DIET FROM LOCALLY AVAILABLE FOODS

In constructing diets it is best to think of four groups of foods:

(1) Staple – Maize, rice, cassava, banana, etc.
(2) Vegetable protein – peas, beans, ground nuts, soya, etc.
(3) Animal protein – milk, eggs, fish, meat.
(4) Dark green vegetables – spinach, cabbage, pumpkin, carrots, etc.

The diet should provide the necessary amounts of the *essential amino acids*. These are the amino acids which cannot be synthesised by the body and must be provided in the food. There are ten essential amino acids, and the deficiency of even one of them will restrict or limit tissue synthesis. The deficient amino acid is termed the 'limiting' amino acid. In general, the limiting amino acid in cereals is lysine and in the legumes it is the sulphur-containing amino acids (SAA) cystine and methionine. The more varied and mixed a diet is, the more are the possibilities that the deficiencies and limitations of one food item will be made good by their presence in an accompanying food. Depending upon the home circumstances, season and availability of foods, an appropriate mixture of the above groups should be suggested, on the general principle that the more mixed and varied the diet, the more balanced it is. Accordingly there will be the following mixtures in order of nutritional adequacy:

(1) Quadrimix   staple/animal protein/vegetable protein/leafy vegetables
(2) Triple Mix   staple/animal protein/vegetable protein
                    staple/animal protein/leafy vegetables
                    staple/vegetable protein/leafy vegetables
(3) Double Mix staple/animal protein
                    staple/vegetable protein
                    staple/leafy vegetables.

Table 2.8 gives the nutrient contents of the commonly used foods in the tropics.

The *quality of protein* in a given mixture is measured by its protein score. It is calculated by comparing the amino acid pattern of the proteins in the food with that of a standard. For practical purposes it is enough to compare the common limiting amino acids lysine and the SAA with the corresponding values in the standard. The standard used is the *reference protein* defined by the joint FAO/WHO Expert Committee on Energy and Protein Requirements. In the reference protein the suggested levels are: lysine 55 mg/1 g protein and SAA 35 mg/1 g protein. Protein score is calculated by first obtaining the quantities in mg/g of protein of these two groups of amino acids from food tables

Table 2.8 Nutrients in commonly used tropical foods

Food	Protein (g/100 g)	Calories (per 100 g)	Limiting amino acids		Per 100 g							
			SAA* (mg/g protein)	Lysine (mg/g protein)	Calcium (mg)	Iron (mg)	Vitamin A potency (i.u.)	Thiamin (mg)	Riboflavin (mg)	Niacin (mg)	Folic acid (mg)	B_{12} (mg)
Egg	13	158	54	59	55	2.8	1000	0.12	0.35	0.1	25	1.7
Chicken	19	139	35	86	15	1.5	Trace	0.10	0.15	9.0	12	Trace
Fish (fresh, lean)	17	73	39	86	20	0.7	–	0.05	0.10	2.5	12	2
Fish (dried, white)	29	125	39	86	40	1.5	–	0.05	0.1	2.5	Trace	Trace
Cow's milk whole	3.3	64	37	80	120	0.1	108	0.04	0.15	0.1	5	0.3
Dried skim milk	36	357	37	80	1260	1.0	Trace	0.45	1.53	1.1	21	3.0
Dried whole milk	25.5	500	37	80	900	0.8	1200	0.30	1.15	0.76	40	2.0
Soya	35	382	30	64	200	7.0	–	1.1	0.3	2.0	–	–
Average legume (e.g. cowpea)	22	340	20	72	90	5.0	20	0.9	0.15	2.0	33	–
Ground nuts (dry)	27	579	20	35	50	2.5	–	0.9	0.15	17.0	110	–
Wheat flour (70% extraction)	10	350	31	21	16	1.5	–	0.08	0.05	0.8	31	–
Rice (polished)	7	352	32	25	5	1.0	–	0.06	0.03	1.0	29	–
Maize (96% extraction)	9.5	362	25	19	12	2.5	150	0.3	0.13	1.5	Trace	–
Millet	9	365	28	21	15	2.0	–	0.2	0.05	1.0	Trace	–
Sorghum	10	353	27	19	20	4.0	–	0.4	0.1	3.0	Trace	–
Oats	12	388	32	27	60	5.0	–	0.5	0.15	1.0	60	–
Potato (Irish)	2	75	26	48	10	0.7	Trace	0.1	0.03	1.5	14	–
Sweet potato	1.5	114	26	48	25	1.0	100	0.1	0.04	0.7	52	–
Taro	2	113	26	48	25	1.0	–	0.1	0.03	1.0	Trace	–
Yam (fresh)	2	104	26	48	10	1.2	–	0.1	0.03	0.4	Trace	–
Plantains	1	128	16	48	7	0.5	20	0.05	0.05	0.7	16	–
Banana	1	116	16	48	7	0.5	100	0.05	0.05	0.7	22	–
Cassava flour	1.5	342	16	48	55	2.0	100	0.04	0.04	0.8	–	–

* Total sulphur-containing amino acids (cystine and methionine).

One International Unit vitamin A = 0.3 μg retinol or 0.6 μg β-carotene (e.g. table 2.8) and then taking the smaller of the two quantities to apply in the formula

$$\text{Protein score} = \frac{\text{Amino acid in mg/g of protein}}{\text{Same amino acid in mg/g of reference protein}} \times \frac{100}{1}$$

For example, to calculate the protein score of wheat, the values of lysine and SAA are obtained from table 2.8 as lysine = 21 mg, SAA = 31 mg. Protein score is calculated using lysine which is the smaller of the two values.

$$\text{Protein score of wheat} = \frac{21}{55} \times 100 = 38.$$

Using this approach, the quality of the protein in the common tropical foods is compared in table 2.9. For adequate nutrition the protein consumed should be of high quality as judged by the protein score, and also should be taken in sufficient amount for the body's needs. If the

Table 2.9 *Protein score of common tropical foods*

Food	Protein score
Egg	154
Chicken	100
Fish	111
Fish (dried, white)	111
Dried skim milk	105
Dried whole milk	105
Soya	85
Average legume	57
Ground nuts	57
Wheat flour (70% extraction)	38
Rice (polished)	45
Maize flour (96% extraction)	34
Millet	38
Sorghum	34
Oats	49
Potatoes	74
Sweet potato	74
Taro, yam	74
Plantain	45
Cassava	45

amount is low, the diet is obviously inadequate; if high, the excess protein is burnt to produce calories and is wasted. These two aspects, *viz.* the quality and quantity factors of dietary protein, are brought together in the concept of Net Dietary protein Calories per cent (NDpCal per cent). The NDpCal per cent can be calculated from the nomogram in figure 2.1. The ideal diet should be adequate in total calories and should provide NDpCal per cent of between 7 and 8. For example, to calculate the NDpCal per cent in a double mix – rice 100 g and legume 10 g, see Table 2.10.

Table 2.10

	Protein (g)	*Calories*	*SAA* (mg)	*Lysine* (mg)
100 g rice =	7.0	352	224	175
10 g legume =	2.2	34	44	158
Total =	9 g	386	268 mg	333 mg

Protein score = $\dfrac{268}{9 \times 35} \times 100 = 85$

Calories derived from protein = 9 x 4 = 36 = 9% of total calories.
From the nomogram figure 2.1, NDpCal per cent = 7.

This double mix, though theoretically correct, may prove impractical. When cooked by boiling the ingredients the bulk may prove too much for a child of, say, 1 year who must eat the amount three times a day. The bulk can obviously be reduced by the addition of edible oil or fat. Fats provide the most concentrated form of calories besides being the source of fat-soluble vitamins, and making the food palatable. The same calories and NDpCal per cent as in the above recipe can be provided by a mixture of rice 70 g, legume 25 g, cooked with 10 g (2 teaspoonsful) of oil.

A major step in nutritional thinking was the realisation that a judicious mix of vegetable protein is theoretically as good as animal protein. The major drawback is the bulk when cooked, so that the calculated volume may exceed the stomach's capacity. The addition of edible oils and oil-containing foods, e.g. ground nuts, soya, coconut and so on, holds the promise of overcoming this difficulty.

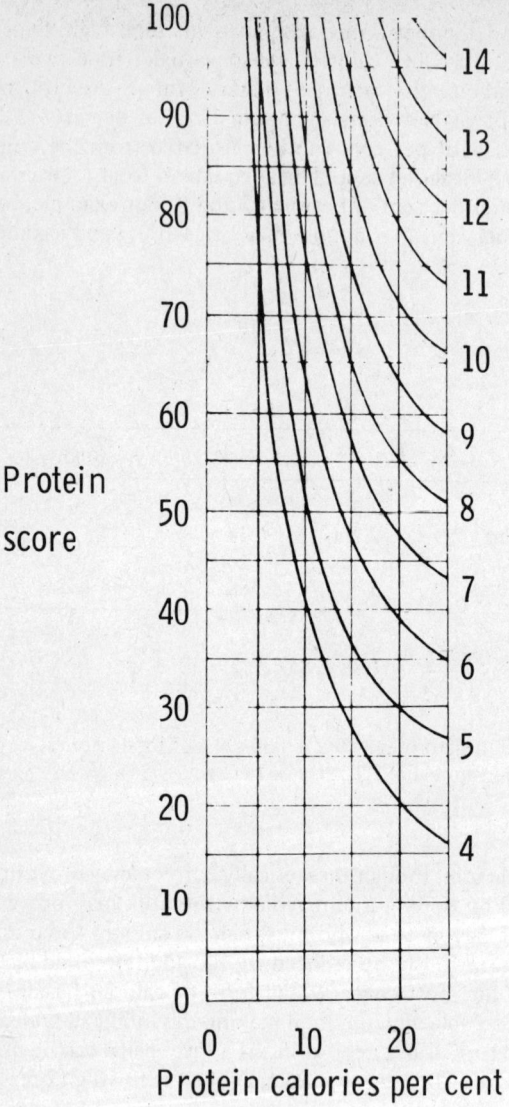

Figure 2.1 Nomogram: net dietary protein calories per cent

FURTHER READING

Food and Agricultural Organization. *Maize and Maize Diets.* FAO Nutrition Studies No. 9. FAO, Rome, 1954.
Food and Agricultural Organization. *Rice and Rice Diets.* FAO Nutrition Studies No. 1. FAO, Rome, 1954.
Food and Agricultural Organization. *Wheat in Human Nutrition.* FAO Nutrition Studies No. 23. FAO, Rome, 1970.
Food and Agricultural Organization. *Legumes in Human Nutrition.* FAO Nutrition Studies No. 19. FAO, Rome, 1973.
Platt, B. S. *Tables of Representative Values of Foods Commonly Used in Tropical Countries.* HMSO, London, 1977.
National Academy of Science. *Tropical Legumes: Resources for the Future.* National Academy of Science, Washington, DC, 1979.
Vogel, S. and Graham, M. *Sorghum and Millet: food production and use.* IDRC-123e. International Development Research Centre, Ottawa, 1979.

Chapter 3

Nutrition in Pregnancy and the Growth of the Fetus

In all mammals, anatomical and physiological changes occur in the body of the mother during pregnancy to create a suitable environment for the growth of the fetus. A complex series of endocrinological and metabolic changes also take place which facilitate the handling of nutrients by the body tissues of the mother as well as their transfer to the fetus. These endocrinological responses provide the basis for the 'metabolic economies' described in the pregnant state. For example, nitrogen balance studies in healthy primigravidae indicate that a positive nitrogen balance is established after week 12. In laboratory rats analyses of body composition at different stages of pregnancy have shown that in early and mid-pregnancy considerable storage of protein occurs. At this time, of course, there are only negligible competitive demands from the fetus. During this phase of anabolism, the increase of muscle nitrogen is about 9 per cent, which is equal to half the amount of nitrogen in the products of conception at term. In late pregnancy, when the fetus is growing rapidly, this protein reserve is called upon so that at parturition no net gain of protein is found. This change to the catabolic phase is induced by the hormones of the growing placenta and occurs irrespective of the protein intake. Thus in rats maternal muscle mass acts as an important reservoir for protein during pregnancy. Similar studies are difficult to conduct in humans, but studies of the amino acid 3-methylhistidine show similar results. This amino acid is liberated during the turnover of protein in muscle, but unlike other amino acids it cannot be utilised and is excreted in urine. The excretion rate rises in late pregnancy, indicating muscle catabolism. These changes in protein metabolism, comprising early conservation followed by utilisation, are similar to those in energy metabolism. Together they help to minimise the effects of inadequate diet during pregnancy on fetal growth.

The fetus is comparatively small in the early stages of pregnancy, even though there is rapid cellular multiplication and differentiation. It is not until the third trimester that fetal growth has reached a stage where nutrients are required in appreciable quantities. Studies in healthy and undernourished women show that, up to the last trimester, there is very little difference in fetal weight between the two groups. Significant changes in weight occur mainly between the twenty-fifth and fortieth weeks of pregnancy.

EFFECTS OF THE PREVIOUS HEALTH AND NUTRITIONAL STATUS OF THE MOTHER

The growth of the fetus can be regarded as a result of the interaction between its genetic potential and the intrauterine environment. Mothers who enter pregnancy in good health, with sound reproductive physiology, and who have not suffered ill-health or nutritional deprivation in childhood, will have larger and healthier infants than mothers who do not have such advantages. Chronic undernutrition in childhood with or without recurrent ill-health is largely responsible for stunting of adult stature. Improvements in health in all the affluent societies of the West are reflected in increase of adult stature. By comparison, the adult female in the developing countries tends to be of short stature and small body build (table 3.1). Thus, there is a significant difference in

Table 3.1 *Average size of the adult female*

	Height (cm)	Weight (kg)
Europe		
United Kingdom	163.6	59.5
Ireland	159.8	61.5
Netherlands	166.3	60.0
Italy	155.4	51.4
France	160.4	55.5
USA	166.5	57.9
Asia		
India	151.7	43.5
Indonesia	150.0	44.0
Phillppines	151.1	48.0
Africa		
Tanzania	150.0	47.7
Ethiopia	152.6	47.0
South America		
Guatemala	142.8	45.7

average birth weights between babies born in affluent societies and those born in the developing countries. Within a society birth weights tend to be higher in the upper socioeconomic groups compared with the lower, and this is in keeping with the differences in several other health indices in the groups (table 3.2). Weight at birth is also influ-

Table 3.2 Birth weight and social class

Place	Population	Subject	Mean birth weight (g)
Madras	Indian	Well-to-do	2985
		Mostly poor	2736
South India	Indian	Wealthy	3182
		Poor	2810
Bombay	Indian	Upper class	3247
		Upper middle class	2945
		Lower middle class	2796
		Lower class	2578
Ghana	African	Prosperous	3188
		General population	2879
Tanzania	African	Upper class	3150
		Lower class	2700
Indonesia	Javanese	Well-to-do	3022
		Poor	2816
Britain	National Cohort 1958	Social class I-II	3380
		Social class V	3290

Source: Tech. Rep. Ser. No. 302, WHO 1965; *J. Trop. Pediat.* (1966), 12, 55; *Br. Med. Bull.* (1981), 37, 260.

enced by factors operating during pregnancy. Serious illnesses, complications of pregnancy, nutritional deprivation, emotional and psychological stress can all influence the growth of the fetus through their adverse effect on the mother, or by interfering with placental growth and transport of nutrients to the fetus.

FETAL GROWTH

Our knowledge of the nutritional requirements for growth in the human fetus has developed from a variety of studies. The relationship between food intake in the mother and its effect on the offspring is best seen in animal experiments, especially in those species where the period of gestation is relatively short and a correlation between dietary intake and fetal growth can be readily seen. There have been epidemiological studies in women comparing birth weights in different social groups, and similar observations during famine and war, which show the effects of acute food shortages on fetal growth. More recently there have been several well-documented studies of nutritional intervention in pregnancy. All such studies indicate that most of the growth in the size of the fetus occurs in the latter part of pregnancy. For example, at the end of the third month of gestation, the fetus weighs approximately 30 g. By comparison, towards the end of gestation the fetus is daily laying down 500 mg of nitrogen (equivalent to 3 g of body tissue), over 300 mg of calcium and 200 mg of phosphorus. The maximum rate of fetal growth is during 32-38 weeks of pregnancy when the weight virtually doubles.

NUTRITIONAL REQUIREMENTS OF THE FETUS

Proteins

The placenta transports protein primarily as amino acids which are then synthesised by the fetus into tissue proteins. Nitrogen balance studies during pregnancy in healthy English women show an average excess of intake over loss of 92 g; since 50 g are needed for the growth of fetal and placental tissues, there is a margin of safety of 42 g, or 45 per cent. By comparison, dietary studies in undernourished Indian women indicate that they have a safety margin of only 6 g, or 12 per cent.

Fat

Most of the 500 g of fetal body fat is deposited between the thirty-fifth and fortieth weeks of pregnancy, about half of this between the thirty-fifth and thirty-eighth weeks. In the early stages of gestation there is no fat laid down apart from essential lipids and phospholipids for the central nervous system and the cell walls. Until the middle of gestation there is only about 0.5 per cent fat in the body of the fetus, after which the amount increases, reaching 7.8 per cent at the thirty-forth week of gestation and 16 per cent before birth. During the last month of intrauterine life as much as 14 g of fat per day is laid down. Of this, placental transport of fatty acids accounts for 40 per cent of fetal fat; the remainder is synthesised by the fetus. Table 2.3 gives the amounts of protein and fat in the normally developing fetus. Both protein and fat increase rapidly in the last 3 months of pregnancy together with the weight of the foetus. Most of the fat is deposited in the subcutaneous tissue so that at term 80 per cent of the body fat is subcutaneous. Fetuses who are small for gestational age have less fat than the larger ones.

Table 3.3 *Protein and fat in the fetal body*

Fetal age (weeks)	12	16	20	24	28	32	36	40
Weight (kg)	0.02	0.1	0.3	0.75	1.35	2.0	2.7	3.5
Protein (g) (derived by N x 6.25)	1.1	6.3	22.5	65	123	189	227	446
Fat (g)	0.1	0.6	2.7	13.1	47.2	120	250	525

Source: Widdowson, E. M. in Dobbing, J. (ed.) *Maternal Nutrition in Pregnancy. Eating for Two?* Academic Press, London, 1981.

Carbohydrate

The fetus has about 9 g of carbohydrate at the thirty-third week of gestation, and at birth it rises to 34 g. The concentration of glycogen in the liver and skeletal muscles increases during the latter part of gestation, as shown in table 3.4. For all nutrients, the fetus and placenta together contain less than 10 per cent of the amounts present in the non-pregnant woman weighing 60 kg.

Table 3.4 *Concentration of carbohydrate (g per 100 g)*

Maturity (weeks)	Heart	Liver	Muscle
31	0.76	0.98	1.63
40	1.01	3.92	2.67

THE ROLE OF THE PLACENTA

The placenta plays an important role in the transfer of nutrients from the mother to the fetus. It is not just an organ of simple transport, but is also able to take up nutrients selectively and either process or resynthesise them before they reach the fetus. The supply of nutrients to the growing fetus depends upon both the amount of maternal blood flowing through the placenta and the food substances carried by it. The efficiency with which the placenta can concentrate, synthesise and transport essential nutrients will also determine the food supply to the fetus.

Factors which regulate fetal growth also regulate the growth of the placenta. Thus the metabolic work of the placenta depends upon the growth capabilities of the fetus and not the other way around. Fetal malnutrition commonly arises either from an insufficient supply from the mother due to some vascular abnormality of the placenta, or from nutritional deficiency in the mother, and only occasionally from reduced placental transport of nutrients. The nature, timing and duration of nutritional deficit is thought to account for the different degrees of intrauterine growth retardation expressed as different forms of fetal malnutrition. It has been estimated that in a third to a half of 'small-for-dates' infants (i.e. with birth weight less than 2500 g) the period of gestation is actually more than 37 weeks; thus, the reduction in birth weight is due to growth-retardation rather than immaturity.

MECHANISM OF PLACENTAL TRANSFER

Various parts of the placenta are actively involved in the transfer, processing and synthesis of nutrients under the influence of maternal, fetal and placental hormones. Gases and water diffuse freely across the placenta, but the mechanism of transport for other substances is not understood. The gradient is not directly from maternal to fetal blood, but from maternal blood to the maternal side of the placenta, where proteins, enzymes, nucleic acids, etc. may be synthesised. Further conversion and synthesis occurs in the fetal part of the placenta (figure 3.1).

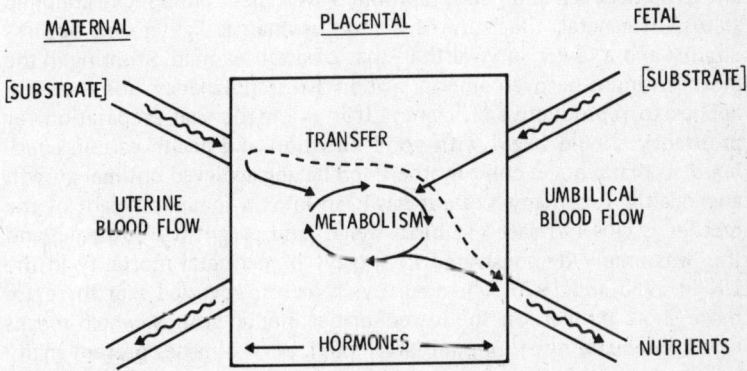

Figure 3.1 Factors affecting transplacental supply of nutrients

Carbohydrate is the principal metabolic fuel of the fetus and is provided in continuous supply by transfer of glucose from the mother through the placenta. On the other hand, fat is not a main source of energy in the fetus, so there is only a slow limited transfer of fatty acids across the placenta. Cell growth in the fetus is assumed to result from fetal synthesis of proteins from the amino acids transferred through the placenta.

Malnourished women, or women in lower socioeconomic groups in developing countries, have a lower mean placental weight compared to well-nourished women or those from higher social groups. In various studies the decrease in mean placental weight has ranged from 14 to 50 per cent. Placentas from malnourished women have reduced DNA content and protein/DNA ratio. Since DNA is a measure of the number of cells in an organ, this indicates that the number of cells in the placentas of malnourished women is reduced. Morphologically there is a reduced villous surface and thus a diminished area for maternal–fetal exchange. The birthweight of a singleton infant correlates significantly with both the wet and dry weight of the placenta.

Heavy infection of the placenta with the malaria parasite can interfere with fetal growth. Chemoprophylaxis with antimalarials during pregnancy will not only ensure adequate placental function but also help protect the mother from anaemia.

NUTRITION OF THE MOTHER

The state of the mother's physiology, especially reproductive physiology, at the time when she commences a pregnancy, has considerable influence on the growth of the fetus. Several studies provide evidence for the relationship between adult size, reproductive efficiency and socioeconomic status. In general, the baby of a short woman is lighter and has less vitality and a lower survival than that of a tall woman. Stunting in the mother cannot be overcome by a good diet in pregnancy, and the same applies to reproductive efficiency. It is axiomatic that preparation for pregnancy should begin with good nutrition and health care in *childhood* so that women enter motherhood having achieved optimal growth and health. For many years it has been known that the height of the mother is closely related to birth weight and pregnancy outcome, and this was amply demonstrated in surveys of perinatal mortality in the UK in 1958 and 1970. These surveys have also revealed that there are more short mothers in the lower socioeconomic groups, which means that inadequate nutrition and larger number of illnesses prevent many girls in this social group from achieving optimal physique. They are thus at a disadvantage as regards childbearing. Similar studies in the United States, conducted by the National Institutes of Health, have shown that mothers who weigh more than 150 lb (68 kg) at conception or who gain more than 30 lb (13.6 kg) in weight during pregnancy tend to have larger and healthier babies with a lower perinatal mortality compared to mothers who weigh less or gain less weight than above.

In addition to the above generalisations there are two factors of special significance for the pregnant woman in the developing world. In all traditional societies marriages occur early, usually around the age of menarche. Hence childbearing also commences early. It is now generally agreed that major risk of low birth weight occurs within 2 years of menarche. For example, the risk of delivering a child less than 2500 g in weight is doubled. Moreover, early childbearing and the resultant competition for nutrients between the fetus and a growing mother, as well as the hormonal changes of pregnancy, may be significant factors in the short stature of women in many developing countries. Secondly, in all traditional societies women have an inferior status. This is reflected in the high mortality rates of infant and young girls compared to boys, a shorter life-expectancy at birth for females as well as higher prevalence rates of nutritional deficiencies in women. Thus the nutrition of the mother during pregnancy is often no different from the deplorable state of nutrition in the non-pregnant woman.

Weight gain in pregnancy

Dietary studies in well-nourished women in Aberdeen showed that the average weight gain during pregnancy was 12.5 kg, including 3.5 kg laid down as fat in the mother, representing an energy store of 30 000 kcal (table 3.5). The gain in weight follows a general pattern:

(1) minimal accumulation (almost all in 'maternal compartment') in the first trimester   1 kg
(2) approximately 0.3 kg per week (of which 60 per cent is in the 'maternal compartment') in the second trimester   3 kg
(3) About 0.3-0.5 kg per week (of which 60 per cent is in the 'fetal compartment') in the third trimester   6 kg

Calorie expenditure is not distributed evenly throughout pregnancy, nor does it parallel fetal growth. Rather it is altered minimally during early gestation, increases sharply near the end of the first trimester and remains fairly constant until term. In the second trimester most of the energy costs are attributed to maternal factors like expansion of blood volume, growth of uterus and breasts, as well as fat storage. In the third trimester most energy costs are for the growth of the fetus and placenta. The total energy cost of pregnancy based on the protein and fat accumulated by the mother and fetus, together with the metabolic cost of accumulation, has been calculated to be 75 000 kcal. Dividing this figure

Table 3.5 *Compartments of weight gain in pregnancy*

Compartment	Cumulative gain (kg) at end of each trimester		
	1	2	3
Fetal compartment			
Fetus	Negligible	1.0	3.4
Placenta	Negligible	0.3	0.6
Amniotic fluid	Negligible	0.4	1.0
Total		1.7	5.0
Maternal compartment			
Increased size of uterus	0.3	0.8	1.0
Increased breast size	0.1	0.3	0.5
Increased blood volume	0.3	1.3	1.5
Increased extracellular fluid	0	0	1.5
Total	0.7	2.4	4.5
Total gain accounted for	0.7	4.1	9.5
Usual gain in weight			12.5 kg
Difference as body fat			3.0 kg

by 250 days yields an increment of 300 kcal/day, equivalent to a 15 per cent increase over non-pregnancy needs.

More recently calorimetric and metabolic studies have provided similar results. The mean daily increase in energy intake in a healthy and well-nourished woman is just over 100 calories for the whole period of pregnancy, with a median value of 9 calories for the first trimester, 84 for the second and 216 for the third. In most cases the addition of 340g of milk to a well-balanced diet is sufficient to meet all the extra energy requirements of pregnancy.

Iron and folic acid requirements

Pregnancy imposes a considerable strain on the maternal blood-forming system. In most instances the greatest need is for iron and to a lesser extent for folic acid. The amount of elemental iron in a fetus at birth is approximately 300 mg and the quantity required for increased red cell formation in the mother to prevent anaemia in the face of increased plasma volume is 500 mg. In other words, the requirement for iron during pregnancy is slightly less than 1 g, concentrated for the most part in the last half of gestation.

In an adequate diet the daily iron content is 10-15 mg, of which 10 -20 per cent is absorbed. Dietary iron will thus provide just a little less than the requirement so that other sources of iron are needed. Body stores of iron, mainly in the bone marrow, are available, but frequently the amount is not sufficient to meet the demand. Iron stores in healthy young American women average 300 mg. However, a significant number of women enter pregnancy with depleted or no iron stores because of previous pregnancies or menstrual loss. The relatively small amounts of iron in the diet, and the low stores of iron, are not enough to meet the greatly increased requirements of iron for the synthesis of maternal and fetal haemoglobin. Thus, anaemia is a relatively common complication of pregnancy, even in developed countries.

Anaemia of pregnancy is common in all developing countries. In a collaborative study involving seven Latin American countries, iron deficiency was present in 48 per cent of pregnant women as compared with 21 per cent of non-pregnant women. Similar prevalence studies have shown that 15-50 per cent of women in Africa, and more than 20 per cent of women in Asia, have haemoglobin levels below 10 g/dl, mostly due to iron deficiency.

Maternal anaemia is associated with an increased risk of low birth weight and perinatal death. In one study in East Africa it was found that among mothers whose haemoglobin was 7.4 g/dl or less at the time of delivery, the incidence of low birth weight ($<$ 2 500 g) was 42 per cent and the stillbirth rate was 147.1 per 1000. In mothers with haemoglobin of 8.8 g/dl and above the incidence of low birth weight was 12.7 per cent and stillbirths 51.0 per 1000. Similarly, in Malaysia it has been reported that in mothers with a haemoglobin of 6.5 g/dl or less the incidence of low birth weight was 20 per cent compared to 7 per cent in non-anaemic pregnancies and the perinatal loss in the anaemic mothers was more than twice that of the non-anaemic ones. More recently a study of 1000 women in India revealed a close relationship between maternal haemoglobin levels and birth weights. 40 per cent of the mothers who gave birth to light infants had haemoglobin levels below 9 g/dl.

Recommended allowances

As described earlier on page 42, studies on the energy costs of pregnancy indicate that about 100 calories per day extra are required for the entire gestation period. These are not evenly distributed but more or less follow the pattern of fetal growth and maternal weight gain. For example, energy balance is maintained by the addition of 10 calories per day in the first trimester, 85 in the second and 220 in the third.

The protein requirement is related to energy intake. Most balance studies show a linear relation between calorie intake and nitrogen balance. The average nitrogen retention during pregnancy is 51±40 mg/kg per day at the average intake of 52±9 calories and 1.7 g protein per kg body weight daily. Based on the above considerations the World Health Organisation has recommended an intake of 1.01 g/kg of protein and 46 kcal/kg for the average woman with a body weight of 55 kg. These recommendations are general and tend to err on the safe side. Most countries have made specific recommendations in relation to their individual circumstances and national dietary patterns (table 2.6).

Table 3.6 Recommended daily protein and energy allowances for women in several countries

Country (year)	Reference body Weight (kg)	Protein (g/kg)		Energy (kcal/kg)	
		Non-pregnant	Pregnant	Non-Pregnant	Pregnant
Canada (1974)	56	0.70	0.85	43	52
Columbia (1955)	55	1.09	1.31	36	40
Guatemala (1969)	55	1.18	2.36	36	40
India (1968)	45	1.00	1.22	49	56
Philippines (1970)	49	1.12	1.32	39	47
United Kingdom (1969)	55	1.00	1.09	40	44
United States (1968)	53	0.95	1.12	34	42

Source: Modified from Calloway, D. H. in M. Winnick (ed.) *Nutrition and Foetal Development*. J. Wiley and Sons, New York, 1976.

As regards iron and folic acid, it has been found that diets which provide the recommended amounts of protein and calories from a mixture of foods will also provide sufficient iron and folic acid. However, to *ensure* adequate intake it is advisable to take additional iron and folic acid, especially in the last trimester.

Effects of nutritional deficiency in pregnancy

Several investigations in laboratory animals show that restricting food in pregnancy can have profound effects on the physiological adjustments in the mother, as well as on the growth and development of the fetus. The effects of restricting only calories cannot be separated from those of restricting proteins, because the body can burn proteins to provide energy; conversely, calories have a protein-sparing effect. Generally speaking, in most laboratory animals food deficiency in pregnancy

Nutrition in Pregnancy and the Growth of the Fetus 45

reduces the size of the litter, the weight of the individual offspring and the survival rate. Subsequent growth of the offspring is also affected, though it is more so when food deficiency extends into the period of lactation.

More recent studies of the cellular mechanisms of growth have measured the DNA content of an organ as an index of cell number and the protein content as an index of cell size. These studies demonstrate that the growth of an organ takes place in phases. There is at first an increase in the number of cells followed by an increase in the size of the individual cell. Food restriction at the time of cell division can significantly affect the size of an organ, and conceivably such a restriction of growth is irreversible.

In the human there are problems in the interpretation of the effects of dietary deficiency on the fetus. In the poorer parts of the world food deficiency during pregnancy is the rule, but comparisons with the more affluent societies are difficult because of the genetic, socioeconomic and other differences. In the case of Western Europe, however, some information is available from 'experiments of nature' like famine and war. During the last war, acute food shortage reaching famine proportions occurred on two separate occasions. The siege of Leningrad lasted 18 months (from August 1941 to January 1943) and for a period of 6 months (September 1941 to February 1942) conditions were extremely severe. Two periods of food deficiency can be identified: a time when there was a generally increasing restriction of food, and, later, a period of *extreme* deficiency when the diet consisted mainly of bread, one half of it made up of defective rye flour and the rest consisting of cellulose, malt and bran. During the early part of the siege the average birth weight decreased significantly. It was found that 49 per cent of those born in the first half of 1942 (thus having suffered nutritional deprivation in the last trimester of pregnancy) weighed less than 2500 g. There were, of course, other potential contributing factors like excessive physical exertion, lack of rest, nervous tension, extremes of cold, and so on.

A similar period of famine was also experienced in Holland in the winter of 1944-45. The period of food shortage was more sharply demarcated than in the case of Leningrad, and overwork and other strains were not so prominent. The famine reached its maximum severity after 6 weeks and lasted for 27 weeks altogether. Thus, pregnant women were exposed to nutritional deprivation for varying lengths of time, but none was exposed for the whole gestation period. Birth weights were lowest in the case of those mothers who had experienced 18-21 weeks of famine, and began to rise immediately after the famine ended. Lowest median birth weights were reached when exposure to famine was in the second half of pregnancy. Exposure very early in pregnancy did not affect the birth weight. Infants born of mothers who had conceived in the latter part of the famine, so that babies experienced 27 weeks of gestation during the famine and an average of 9 weeks after it ended, attained a higher mean birth weight than those born in the early part of the famine.

In the developing world, food shortage is chronic and is often acute during times of poor harvests. In a dietary survey of 352 pregnant women in India, it was found that the mean daily intake was 1402 kcal and 38 g protein. (WHO/FAO recommended allowances are 2200 cal and 55 g protein.) Many women in the lower socioeconomic groups enter pregnancy after a childhood in which undernutrition and recurrent illnesses are common, so that they have not obtained the optimum in growth and physiological development. Thus, the mean body weight in 498 non-pregnant Indian women in the low socioeconomic group was found to be only 42.4 kg; 40 per cent of women in the low and low-middle income groups in India are under 150 cm in height whereas only 15-20 per cent in the upper income groups are of short stature, again indicating the importance of nutrition in early childhood. Moreover, on their marginal nutrition many pregnant women gain very little weight. In one study of 48 pregnant women, the mean gain in body weight from the twelfth to the fortieth week of pregnancy was 6.02 kg. In another study of 130 pregnant women, almost half failed to gain weight between the thirty-second and thirty-sixth weeks and thereafter. Besides poor weight-gain, many show clinical signs of nutritional deficiency. In a nutritional survey carried out amongst 198 pregnant women during the third trimester of pregnancy, 44 per cent showed clinical signs of vitamin B complex deficiency, 9.5 per cent had oedema of the legs and 14.5 per cent showed signs of lack of vitamin A. The mean birth weight in such women from the lower socioeconomic group was 2778 g as compared to 3055 g in the higher social group.

A survey of dietary intake of women in coastal Tanzania revealed that mean daily energy intake was 1850 kcal and that of protein was 51.5 g. Iron intake in the diet ranged from 10 to 16.2 mg per day. A significant correlation was seen between the energy intake of the mother and the size of the baby. In order to have a baby weighing more than 3.1 kg it was necessary that the mother should consume at least 50 g of protein daily. Forty per cent of the women were eating less protein than this amount. Energy deficiency was a much more serious problem. To have a baby weighing 3.1 kg a mother had to consume 2200 cal per day, and only 20 per cent of the women had as much.

A similar study in four Guatemalan villages showed that the mean intake of calories and protein during pregnancy was 1500 cal and 40 g respectively. The average maternal height in rural Guatemala is 143 cm which is far less than the average height for women in a sample of the white population in the USA. Much of this low maternal height is accounted for by growth retardation during the first 7 years of life. The average weight gain in pregnancy was 7 kg, which is about half of that in well-nourished women in affluent societies. Predictably, the mean birth weight was low at 3 kg and of 39 infants with normal gestational age about a third weighed 2.5 kg or less. Dietary histories again indicated a close association between food intake and the weight of the baby at birth. For example, in 34 women with a daily caloric intake of 700-1800, the mean birth weight was 2.8 kg. In eight women with a daily caloric intake of 1900 to 2,100 calories the mean birthweight was 3 kg and in 9 women with a daily caloric intake of 2200 - 3100 calories the mean birth weight was 3.2 kg. Supplementation studies showed that the total caloric intake was a more critical variable than protein, and the incidence of lighter babies was highest when the Guatemalan mother consumed less than 1800 cal per day.

In peasant societies the wet season is often the worst time of the year. Food shortages, heavy demands for agricultural work, increased exposure to infection like malaria, diarrhoea and respiratory infection, all coincide to increase stress and poverty. Malnutrition, sickness and indebtedness more commonly occur in the rainy season. Naturally, the weaker groups like mothers and children suffer most. Pregnancies which reach the advanced stage in the wet season are at special risk of resulting in low-birth weight infants. The greatest demand is made on the adult population by the energy expenditure needed for farming. For example, in Upper Volta it was noticed that energy expenditure by women in the wet season was between 2450 and 3600 kcal compared to 2000-2700 in the dry season.

CELLULAR GROWTH IN THE FETUS

The organ sizes and body weights of infants who were either stillborn or died in the neonatal period, were compared in the case of 1002 consecutive necropsies in New York City. In the case of mothers from the low socioeconomic groups, the body size of the infants - as well as the weights of the brain, heart, liver, spleen, thymus, kidneys and adrenals - were all significantly less than in the case of infants born to better-off mothers. The body weight was less by 13-17 per cent of the mean of infants born to well-to-do mothers. Amongst the organs, the thymus, spleen and liver were found to be particularly small.

Measurements of DNA and DNA to protein ratio in kidney, heart and liver of the human fetus indicate that these organs grow in several phases during intruterine life:

(1) Between the fourteenth and twenty-fifth week of intrauterine life,

the cells in all the three organs are dividing rapidly. The DNA content approximately doubles each week.
(2) Between the thirtieth and fortieth weeks there is a rapid growth in cell size. The cells still increase in number, but more slowly than before.
(3) At term all three organs still had less than 20 per cent of the numbers of cells characteristic of the adult, indicating that further increase in cell number occurs after birth.

In the case of babies who were 'small-for-dates' the protein/DNA ratio was normal, but the *total* DNA tended to be low.

WEIGHT AT BIRTH AND BODY COMPOSITION OF THE FETUS

When the body composition of stillborn infants in undernourished Indian women was compared with that of similar infants of well-nourished English women, it was found that at 26-28 weeks of gestation the total body weights were similar in both groups, but there were significant qualitative differences. There was a deficit in protein and iron content in the case of the Indian babies (Table 3.7). In the case of Indian fetuses, liver stores of vitamin A, B_2 and folate were lower than those of infants of well-nourished mothers.

Table 3.7 *Fetal body composition in undernourished Indian and healthy English women at different weights and gestational age.*

	Age (weeks)	Water (g)	Protein (g)	Fat (g)	Cu (g)	Po_4 (g)	Mg (mg)	Iron (mg)
Weight 1000 g								
Indian[a]	27	862	80	26	5.8	3.3	200	59
English[b]	26	860	87.5	10	60	3.4	220	64
Weight 1500 g								
Indian	34	1248	126	75	10.5	5.0	325	81
English	31	1270	156	35	10.0	5.6	350	100
Weight 2000 g								
Indian	38	1604	176	148	14.6	8.6	425	108
English	33	1620	231	100	15.0	8.2	460	160
Weight 2500 g								
Indian	40	1935	242	242	19.0	10.8	540	138
English	35	1940	306	185	20	11	580	220
Weight 3000 g								
Indian	40	2238	291	366	22.7	11.4	655	165
English	38	2180	344	360	25.0	14.0	700	260

[a] Apte, S. and Iyengar, L. *Br. J. Nutr.* (1972), 27, 305.
[b] Widdowson, E. M. in N. S. Assali (ed.), *Biology of Gestation*, vol. 2, Academic Press, N.Y.

EFFECTS OF SUPPLEMENTING MATERNAL DIET

In well-nourished communities no supplementation is necessary beyond the administration of iron and folic acid in the last trimester and the normal satisfaction of hunger from a mixed diet. In communities where diets are inadequate, and where a large proportion of mothers enter reproduction after a childhood characterised by inadequate growth, supplementation is important to avoid fetal malnutrition. Repeated pregnancies in such a situation lead to depletion of maternal tissues and impaired reproductive efficiency.

Several countries have now evolved national programmes for protecting the diets of pregnant and lactating women through a supply of free subsidised foods, especially milk; through the establishment of fair-price retail shops; through fortification of ordinary foods to improve their nutritive value; and sometimes through cash benefits to improve purchasing power.

In developing countries, where health resources are meagre and a large number of families exist on marginal nutrition, it is necessary to identify the minimum supplementation necessary for adequate fetal growth. It is now generally agreed that maternal weight gain in pregnancy is associated with fetal growth. Generally, 1 kg of maternal weight gain leads to an increment of 20–25 g in the birth weight. More specifically, a weekly weight gain of less than 0.2 kg more than doubles the likelihood of the incidence of low birth weight. The effect is even more serious if the pre-pregnancy weight was at the lower end of the scale. The correlation of birth weight with the post-partum weight of the mother is even closer. In several studies mean birth weight has been shown to increase linearly with the post-partum weight until the post-partum weight is 100–110 per cent of ideal maternal weight. At that point birth weight remains constant while post-partum weight continues to increase.

The above studies suggest that fetal growth occurs optimally only when the mother is able to accumulate a critical amount of extra body stores during pregnancy. Thus the metabolic adaptations of pregnancy enable the mother initially to maintain her own body stores of nutrients. If she has adequate quantities of these stores she can succeed in supporting a normal rate of fetal growth even if her own food intake becomes inadequate. If the body stores are small, then the level of food intake seems crucial for maintaining a normal rate of growth in the fetus.

Studies in Guatemala have shown that supplementing the pregnant woman's diet by 233 kcal per day led to a significant increase in fetal birth weight. Heavier babies were born to mothers who consumed more calories during pregnancy, irrespective of whether the calories were derived from the usual diet or from food supplements. The conversion of food calories into fetal tissues was at the rate of 3 g of baby per 1000 kcal of additional food. It was significant that in the same mother there was an average difference of 2.2 g between successive siblings per change of 1000 kcal in the diet. Though there are a host of factors which can influence birthweight, these findings emphasise the importance of adequate food intake during pregnancy. The association between weight gain in pregnancy and birth weight, though statistically significant, is not very strong. Correlation coefficient has been between 0.2 and 0.3 in most studies, and weight gain in pregnancy accounts for about 6 per cent of the variance for birth weights. However, what is more important is the shift of emphasis from protein to calories. In most instances, when the energy requirement is satisfied by adequate food intake, the requirement of protein is also taken care of, unless the diet is bizarre.

More recent work in India adds yet another facet to the whole question of supplementation in pregnancy. When diets of Indian women in low socio-economic groups were supplemented with 50 g protein and 500 cal, the mean gain in weight by the mothers during pregnancy was 2.84 kg, significantly greater than the 1.02 kg in the control group; the mean birth weight of the babies (3000 g) was also significantly greater than that of the controls (2700 g). Interestingly, when the supplement consisted of 30–60 mg of iron and 200–500 mg of folic acid, instead of food, the mean birth weight was 2880 g compared to 2500 g in the controls and the incidence of babies weighing less than 2300 g was 10 per cent as compared to 23 per cent in the control group. The placentas in the supplemented group were heavier and their DNA content was higher. It has been suggested that folic acid has a growth-promoting action besides being a haemopoietic factor. On the basis of these studies the government of India has commenced a national programme of supplementation with iron and folic acid for pregnant women.

INTERVENTION PROGRAMMES

In the past decade several carefully documented studies in pregnant women have demonstrated the importance of adequate dietary intake for optimal fetal growth. For example, in *Montreal* it was found that pregnant women who were referred for dietary intervention delivered infants with mean birth weights 40 g heavier than in the controls. The frequency of low birth weight was 5.7 per cent among those referred compared to 6.8 per cent in controls. Compared to their matched controls, primigravidae had a 61 g advantage and women who weighed less than 64 kg at conception had a 63 g advantage. Women who were both primigravidae and weighed less than 64 kg had a 73 g advantage. In rural *Guatemala* where the daily diet consisted of 1500 cal and 40 g protein, the proportion of infants born with low birth weight (<2500 g) was 20 per cent. A daily supplement of 70 cal resulted in a gain of 56 g in birth weight. These and similar other studies referred to in the preceding discussion indicate that in women at risk of low birth weight, food supplementation in pregnancy can lead to an increase of between 40 and 60 g in birth weight. The degree of rise depends on the nutritional status of the woman. In thin and undernourished women the rise in birth weight is most evident. In starved women, as for example during the Dutch famine, a deficit of 300–400 g can be made up almost immediately upon adequate feeding.

There is an urgent need to convert the above information into viable health programmes. It is estimated that of the 22 million babies being born with a birth weight less than 2500 g each year, 21 million are in the developing world. A high proportion of neonatal and infant mortality in the developing countries occurs in such infants, so that the effects of fetal malnutrition work well into the first year of life. Moreover, in all countries the incidence of handicaps is also higher in infants with low birth weight compared to normal.

The mean birth weight in the community, and especially the ratio between mean birth weights in the lower and upper socioeconomic groups, is increasingly recognised as a useful measure of the nutrition of the community. This is more so because of the inferior status of the woman in many traditional societies. All intervention programmes have the tendency to follow the Inverse Care Law and benefit the upper strata of the community more than the needy ones. Serial improvements in mean birth weight, and particularly in the proportion of those born with a birth weight less than 2500 g, serve as readily available indices of community nutrition. They also serve as measures of the effectiveness with which nutrition programmes reach the disadvantaged such as, for example, women in the lower socioeconomic groups.

All interventions reach the consumer through services. Hence prenatal care becomes a priority where nutrition in pregnancy is concerned. In developing countries not more than a third of the pregnant women receive any antenatal care, and the number of women receiving skilled assistance in labour is even smaller. National health programmes in most countries have continued to emphasise institutional care at the cost of coverage with basic services so that improvements in health and nutrition status have been disappointing. For example, in Hyderabad (India) studies undertaken in the 1960s showed that the daily energy intake of pregnant women in low socioeconomic groups was between 1400 and 1600 kcal. A decade later, in spite of several socioeconomic improvements as well as expansion of education and health-care delivery in urban areas, dietary intakes have remained essentially similar to those of two decades ago. Moreover, the mean body weights during the third trimester of pregnancy (49.5 kg) and mean weight gain in pregnancy (6 kg) have remained unaltered over the past 15 years. Thus, the considerable amount of new scientific knowledge and experience of the past two decades has not benefited the large majority of the population. Radical new approaches in developing health-care strategy to expand coverage with basic services are needed.

All innovative approaches aimed at extending health coverage have tended to utilise traditional health providers in the community. Several countries, notably Sudan, Niger, Tanzania, Indonesia, Malaysia and the Philippines, have new national programmes for training traditional birth attendants and their subsequent deployment as village midwives. Such health workers may succeed in improving traditional food habits, and can become a local source of nutritional advice as well as distribution of iron and folic acid tablets, and antimalarials where necessary, to the pregnant women. But there is also a need of interventions at other levels through programmes of education, especially female literacy, creation of job opportunities, and availability of subsidised food items for the pregnant woman.

Greater awareness of the nutritional needs of the pregnant woman in the community must be accompanied by development of local skills and facilities for monitoring adequate fetal growth. Here measurements of sequential fundal height and abdominal girth as measures of fetal growth have been evaluated in several studies and can be developed into a simple tool for use in villages and peri-urban communities. The trained birth attendant can thus help in the primary and secondary selection of pregnant women for more expert care.

FURTHER READING

Brozek, J., Coursin, D. B. and Read, M. S. Longitudinal studies on the effects of malnutrition, supplementation and behavioural stimulation. *Bull. Pan Am. Hlth. Org.*, (1977), **11**, 237-49.

Chavez, A. and Martinez, C. The effect of maternal supplementation on infant development. *Arch. Latinoamer. Nutr.* (1979), **29**, 143-53.

Naismith, D. J. Diet during pregnancy − a rationale for prescription. In Dobbin, J. (ed.) *Maternal Nutrition in Pregnancy − eating for two?* Academic Press, London and New York, 1981.

Rush, D. Nutritional services during pregnancy and birth weight: a retrospective matched pair analysis. *Can. Med. Assoc. Jl.* (1981), **125**, 567-76.

Stein, Z., Susser, M. and Saenger, G. *Famine and Human Development: the Dutch Hunger Winter of 1944/45.* Oxford University Press, New York, 1975.

Villar, J., Belizan, J. M. and Delgado, H. Monitoring foetal growth in rural areas: an alternative utilising non-professional personnel. *Bull. Pan. Am. Hlth. Org.* (1979), **13**, 117-23.

Widdowson, E. M., Southgate, D. A. T. and Hey, E. N. Body composition of the fetus and infant. In Visser, H. K. A. (ed.) *Nutrition and Metabolism of the Fetus and Infant.* Proceedings of the 5th Nutricia Symposium. pp.167-77. Martinus Nijhoff, The Hague, 1979.

Winick, M. (ed.) *Current Concepts in Nutrition*, vol. 3, pp. 127-46. John Wiley & Sons, New York, 1974.

Chapter 4

Breast Feeding

All babies thrive on their mother's milk. The period of neonatal life and early infancy is characterised by rapid growth, so that the average baby at 4 months of life weighs twice as much as at birth, and three times as much when 12 months old. This increase in growth includes increased muscle mass, growth of organs, expansion of blood volume and linear increase in the long bones. The nutrients required to sustain such a rapid growth are all supplied by breast milk alone in the first 3-4 months of life, in all infants. The composition of human milk should therefore provide a clue to the physiological needs for energy and nutrients in infants.

PROTEIN REQUIREMENTS

Various studies have been conducted to ascertain the requirements of protein during infancy. In one type of study, infants were fed mixtures of amino acids in different combinations and the levels of individual amino acids which supported adequate growth were taken as the optimal levels. In another study, infants were fed a variety of milk formulae in quantities which maintained adequate growth and the concentration of each individual amino acid in the milk was then calculated to give the required amount. Using the data from these studies an Expert Committee of the World Health Organisation made recommendations on the amino acid requirements in infants (table 4.1).

In adults, eight amino acids are essential. They cannot be synthesised in the body and must be supplied in food. These are isoleucine, leucine, lysine, methionine, phenylalanine, threonine, tryptophan and valine. Infants require these eight plus histidine. Precise information on the requirements of amino acids at different periods of growth in the infant is lacking. Based on studies of intake of breast milk in Swedish infants and the composition of human milk, the above information about

Table 4.1 *Estimated requirements of essential amino acids*

Amino acid	Amino acid mixture which will maintain adequate growth (mg/kg/day)[a]	Amino acid content of various milk formulae which will maintain adequate growth (mg/kg/day)[b]	Suggested pattern (mg/g protein)[c]	Pattern in breast milk (mg/g protein)[d]
Histidine	34	28	14	31
Isoleucine	119	70	35	67
Leucine	229	161	80	120
Lysine	103	161	52	90
Methionine and cystine	45 + cystine	58	29	44
Phenylalanine and tyrosine	90 + tyrosine	125	63	86
Threonine	87	116	44	58
Tryptophan	22	17	8.5	30
Valine	105	93	47	87

[a] Holt, L. E. and Syderman, S. E. in W. L. Nyah (ed.) *Amino Acid Metabolism and Genetic Variation*, p. 381. McGraw-Hill, New York, 1967.
[b] Fomon, S. J. and Filer, L. J.
[c] Joint FAO/WHO Expert Committee, 1973.
[d] Based on 100 ml of breast milk = 1.07 g protein. *DHSS Report on Health and Social Subjects*, No. 12 HMSO, London, 1977.

average daily intake of various amino acids at different ages can be derived (table 4.2).

Amino-acid pattern

Besides the total quantity of amino acids present, the proportion in which they occur is also important with regard to the utilisation of a protein food. The relationship of each individual amino acid to other amino acids determines the efficiency of its utilisation by the body. Hence the *pattern* of amino acids in food is one of the important factors influencing the total amount of protein required. Each individual protein has its own turnover rate, responding in a specific way to any change in metabolism. The turnover in the whole body is the result

Table 4.2 *Estimated daily intake of energy, protein and essential amino acids at different ages in breast-fed infants*

	1 month	2 months	3 months	6 months
Mean intake of breast milk (ml)	600	727	765	780
Calories	420	509	535	546
Protein (g)	6.4	7.7	8.2	8.3
Amino acids (mg)				
Histidine	186	225	237	241
Isoleucine	402	487	512	522
Leucine	720	872	918	936
Lysine	540	654	688	702
Methionine	114	138	145	148
Phenylalanine	288	348	367	374
Threonine	348	421	443	452
Tryptophan	180	218	229	234
Valine	522	632	655	678

Table 4.3 *Comparison of patterns of amino acid requirements with that of milk and egg proteins (mg per g of protein)*

Amino acid	Suggested pattern of requirements[a]	Composition of protein		
		Human milk[b]	Cow's milk	Egg
Histidine	14	29	27	22
Isoleucine	35	62	47	54
Leucine	80	112	95	86
Lysine	52	84	78	70
Methionine and Cystine	29	41	33	57
Phenylalanine and Tyrosine	63	80	102	93
Threonine	44	54	44	47
Tryptophan	8.5	28	14	17
Valine	47	81	64	66

[a] Joint FAO/WHO Expert Committee, 1973.
[b] *DHSS Report on Health and Social Subjects*, No. 12. HMSO, London, 1977.

of these activities. Feeding studies in infants show that the pattern of amino acids found most suitable for supporting growth also resembles closely the pattern found in breast milk. Table 4.3 compares the patterns of requirement in infants with those of breast milk, cow's milk and egg proteins. It is obvious from the table that the protein of breast milk will be utilised with the greatest efficiency by the infant.

Human milk has a high concentration of free amino acids equivalent to a fifth of total milk nitrogen compared with 5 per cent in cow's milk and most milk formulae. Moreover, amongst the amino acids of human milk, free taurine is prominent, in contrast to its low concentration in cow's milk and its virtual absence from formula feeds. Infants cannot synthesise taurine from cysteine, which should be a matter of concern in view of the high concentration of taurine found in the developing central nervous system of the newborn in many species including man.

Metabolism of milk protein

Do the quality and quantity of protein in the infant's diet affect his well-being in any way? Present evidence suggests that it is almost certainly so in the case of the low birth weight infant and very likely so in the case of the normal newborn. In the pre-term infant many of the enzyme systems in the liver are not fully developed. For example, the mechanism for making cystine from methionine is incomplete in the pre-term baby, so that unlike the adult, he must rely on an exogenous supply of cystine. Cow's milk is a poor source of cystine and infants fed on cow's milk-based formulae are likely to experience a deficiency of this amino acid. In the same way, the capacity for the *breakdown* of amino acids is impaired in pre-term infants, especially with regard to phenylalanine and tyrosine. When these babies are fed cow's milk-based formulae, with high protein concentrations, the blood levels of these two amino acids rise, reaching in some cases levels as high as those in phenylketonuria. Furthermore, these high blood concentrations are known to persist for as long as 6 weeks. Hence, from this point of view alone, there are several risks in the artificial feeding of infants; these are greater in the pre-term infant or in the infant whose physiological reserves have been compromised by asphyxia, trauma, infection or congenital defects. With regard to amino acid composition, the two main characteristics of human milk are the low ratio between methionine and cystine, and the relatively low content of the amino acids phenylalanine and tyrosine. In fact, the protein of human milk is the only known animal protein with a methionine/cystine ratio less than 1.0. Only vegetable proteins demonstrate this property.

Milk fat

The fat in milk is the main source of energy since, per unit weight, it provides twice the amount of energy derived from either protein or sugar.

Naturally occurring fatty acids contain 4 to 24 carbon atoms in a molecule. According to the number of carbon atoms present, they are divided into long (18 or more carbon atoms), medium (8 to 12 carbon atoms), and short (4 to 6 carbon atoms) chain fatty acids. The short chain fatty acids are not abundant in food fats. The medium chain acids are also not very common, but are of interest because they are absorbed through the portal circulation instead of the intestinal lymphatics. Long chain fatty acids constitute the major proportion of fat in both human and cow's milk.

The fatty acids are also classified as saturated or unsaturated, depending upon the presence of double bonds between the carbon atoms. The unsaturated ones may be mono- or poly-unsaturated, depending upon the number of carbon atoms with double bonds. As a general rule, the absorption of fatty acids in the gut is inversely related to the number of carbon atoms. The *longer* the chain, the less efficient is the absorption. On the other hand, the *more* the number of double bonds, the better the absorption.

In all milks the fat contains mainly long chain acids with 14 to 22 carbon atoms. Depending upon the species, the fatty acids occur in varying quantities of saturated and unsaturated ones. An important consideration in the synthesis of milk fat in the cow is the rumen, which acts as a large fermentation tank with a capacity of several gallons, depending upon the size of the animal. Cellulose is broken down in the rumen by the action of bacteria and protozoa and the products of this fermentation, like acetate, butyrate, etc., are utilised in the synthesis of lipids. Hence cow's milk contains a large proportion of short chain fatty acids. Moreover, the lipids within the rumen, being plant lipids, are highly unsaturated when they are first released from their vegetable source. They then undergo rapid hydrogenation in the fermenting environment of the rumen and are converted into saturated fats. These are then absorbed and contribute to the saturated fatty acids of milk. In contrast, the fat in human milk consists mainly of unsaturated fatty acids.

Milk fat is an important source of energy and the fat-soluble vitamins. The breast-fed infant is able to absorb more than 90 per cent of the ingested fat at the age of 1 week, compared to 70 per cent of the fat in cow's milk or the fat from proprietary formulae containing a mixture of animal and vegetable fats. The absorption of fat becomes more

Table 4.4 Fat content of human and cow's milk per 100 ml milk

	Fat (g)	Cholesterol (mg)	Energy (kcal)	Total saturated fatty acids (mg)	Total mono-unsaturated fatty acids (mg)	Total poly-unsaturated fatty acids (mg)
Human milk mean (Range)	4.2 (3.7–4.8)	16 (12–23)	70 (65–75)	2001	1612	317
Cow's milk	3.9	14	67	2330	1244	107

Table 4.5 The concentration of different fatty acids in human and cow's milk (mg/100 ml milk)

Fatty acid		Human milk	Cow's milk
Butyric	4 : 0	0	118
Caporic	6 : 0	0	74
Caprylic	8 : 0	Trace	44
Capric	10 : 0	54	103
Lauric	12 : 0	213	129
Myristic	14 : 0	290	413
Palmitic	16 : 0	1051	959
Stearic	18 : 0	393	413
Others		Trace	77
Total saturated		2001	2330
Myristoleic	14 : 1	Trace	52
Palmitoleic	16 : 1	160	100
Oleic	18 : 1	1408	1026
Others		44	66
Total mono-unsaturated		1612	1244
Linoleic	18 : 2	285	52
Linolenic	18 : 3	32	55
Arachidonic	20 : 4	Trace	Trace
Others		Trace	Trace
Total poly-unsaturated		317	107

efficient as the infant gets older, but even at the age of 1 month, breast milk fat is absorbed better than that in cow's milk.

The fatty acid composition of breast milk is dependent upon the source of fat in the mother's diet, and the total quantity of fat varies according to the adequacy of calories and other nutrients. Lipid content is also dependent upon the presence or otherwise of depot fat and its availability for the synthesis of milk fat. Thus, fatty acids of human milk are unique to each individual mother. Nonetheless, one can recognise a constant pattern in the lipids of human milk. When breast milk from mothers in different countries was analysed, it was found that the most important difference lay in short chain fatty acids with 10 to 14 carbon atoms. These acids were in higher concentration in East African and Asian mothers. The high proportion of C10 to C14 acids was associated with a relatively lower proportion of C16 to C18 acids in both the saturated and unsaturated groups. This is probably due to the fact that Europeans live on a high-fat diet rich in C16 to C18 acids and the mammary gland has little need to synthesise new fatty acids. The East African communities use foods which are low in fat, and the high proportion of C10 to C14 acids in their milk is due to net synthesis within the breast of fat from carbohydrate sources.

When specimens of tissue fat in infants are analysed for their fatty acid composition, it is found that the nature of body fat is largely determined by that of the dietary fat. Infants fed on human milk have a different composition of tissue fat from those fed on cow's milk or on milk formulae containing vegetable oils. This observation is important for two reasons. The brain and the rest of the nervous system undergo rapid growth throughout early infancy. Though the brain cells are largely developed by the time of birth, myelin is still to be laid along the axons and the dendritic connections. Fat is an important constituent of myelin, as indeed of the rest of the nervous system. The accumulation of long chain polyunsaturated fatty acids (C20 and above) in the developing brain starts before birth. It continues after birth and myelination is not complete until about 4 years of age. The tissues of the newborn infant are capable of synthesising these long chain fatty acids from their precursors, chiefly linoleic (C18:2) and linolenic acids (C18:3). The brain appears to have a priority for the precursors when supplies are short. Animal experiments indicate that the brain lipids are altered according to diets fed to the newborn. There is no proof as yet that this is also the case in the human, but the results of animal experiments suggest that this cannot be ruled out. Thus, intake of biologically inappropriate fatty acids could produce a long-lasting effect on the growth of the nervous system. Secondly, as far as the intake of nutrients is concerned, the infant is dependent upon just one food source, milk. Unlike the adult who eats a varied diet and has several food sources providing a rich variety of nutrients, the infant's choice is restricted to those nutrients which are present in the milk with which he is being fed. There is virtually no margin of safety and any inadequacy in the milk will be translated into altered composition of body tissues being formed at the time. Such a deficiency is then likely to be carried over to a future period when the required nutrients become available and the deficiency can be corrected. Whether such a restructuring of myelin can occur is not yet known, but present evidence suggests that it is unlikely because of the very slow turnover rate of myelin.

In order to avoid this difficulty, the manufacturers of many brands of powdered milks modify the fat composition by removing butter fat from cow's milk and replacing it with vegetable oils (Table 4.4, 4.5 and

Table 4.6 *Fatty acid composition of human and cow's milk[a], several proprietary infant feeding formulae[a] and commonly used vegetable fats[b] in their manufacture*

Fatty acids	Saturated					Unsaturated			
	$C10:0$	$C12:0$	$C14:0$	$C16:0$	$C18:0$	$C16:1$	$C18:1$	$C18:2$	$C18:3$
Human milk	1.3	5	7	25	9.3	3.8	33	6.7	<1
Cow's milk	2.7	3.3	10.8	25	10.8	2.6	27	1.3	1.4
SMA	1	10	6	16	11	1	29	24	2
Nativa	2	9	9	22	7	1	35	13	1
Almiron B	0	0	<1	11	2	<1	27	58	2
Farilacid	2	2	9	25	14	2	35	7	1
Frisolac	<1	6	3	32	4	0	38	16	0
Similac	2	19	7	9	3	0	19	40	<1
Milumil	1	4	7	35	8	1	32	10	0
Nan	2	4	11	31	9	2	24	16	1
Pelargon	2	2	8	24	11	1	30	16	1
Humana 1 and 2	1	7	4	23	8	<1	44	13	<1
Oleo oils	–	0.2	3.3	26	20	–	45.5	3.0	0.5
Corn oil	–	–	–	13	4	–	29.0	54.0	–
Coconut oil	6	49.5	19.5	8.5	2	–	6.0	1.5	–
Soya oil	–	–	Trace	11.0	4	–	25.0	51.0	9.0
Cottonseed oil	–	–	1.0	29.0	4	2	24.0	40.0	–

[a] Expressed as g/100 g total fat.
[b] Expressed as g/100 g of the oil.

4.6). This practice gives rise to even more difficulties. For example, when infants were offered feeds in which 60 per cent of the fatty acids were in the form of linoleic (C18:2) acid, a rapid increase in the amount of linoleic acid in the adipose tissue was noted. Such a change is accompanied by alteration in the phospholipid composition of cell membranes, especially of the erythrocytes. It was found that in pre-term babies fed infant formulae rich in poly-unsaturated fatty acids, the erythrocyte cell membrane becomes at risk of peroxidation. Iron added to the formulae generates free radicals which initiate the process of peroxide haemolysis of the erythrocyte. To avoid this, large amounts of vitamin E (an antioxidant) are needed.

Several reports on the antiviral properties of human milk have been published, and are discussed in the sections which follow. It has been shown that the lipid component of milk and colostrum has pronounced antiviral action against all dengue types of viruses as well as Japanese B encephalitis; St Louis encephalitis; West Nile, yellow fever, Herpes hominis and polio viruses. A strong relationship between lipase activity in milk and antimicrobial activity was demonstrated leading to the identification of monoglycerides and fatty acids as the active agents. Human milk has high lipase activity which helps fat digestion and the release of fatty acids and monoglycerides.

Carbohydrate

Lactose is the predominant sugar in the milk of most mammals, with very few exceptions. The extremes of variation in the lactose content of the milk of mammals are from 4 g per dl in the dog and the elephant to about 7 g per dl in man. By contrast, the fat composition can vary by almost 30-fold. This relative constancy of lactose secretion in milk is an indication of its important role in mammalian biology. The nature of this role needs to be determined, but for the present one can speculate along the following lines:

(1) Amongst the various sugars, per molecule (and hence per unit of osmotic pressure) lactose provides twice the calorific value of glucose. Since milk is secreted at the same osmotic pressure as plasma, there is less energy consumed in maintaining osmotic equilibrium when lactose is used as the main sugar. In human milk, lactose accounts for half the osmotic pressure, the remainder being due to monovalent ions like Na^+, K^+, Cl^-, etc. Because of the high concentration of lactose in breast milk, the solute content of breast milk is low, which makes it well suited for the immature kidneys of the infant.

(2) High concentration of lactose in human milk influences the pH of the gut in the newborn and its bacterial flora. Together with other immune factors to be described below, the high lactose concentration of breast milk prevents the growth of the potentially dangerous pathogen, *Escherichia coli*, and instead promotes colonisation by *Lactobacillus*.

(3) It is likely that lactose is utilised for the synthesis of the galactolipids of the growing brain in the infant. In many mammalian species the quantity of galactose per unit weight of brain tissue of the offspring is closely related to the lactose content of the mother's milk. However, children suffering from galactosaemia or lactose intolerance who receive diets free of galactose and lactose for many years since infancy have not shown any obvious ill effects. It has been pointed out that the glycolipids, glycoproteins and glycoaminoglycans of the central nervous system can be synthesised from glucose in the liver. Cow's milk is low in lactose; and so, in the manufacture of many infant feeding formulae, the first stage in the 'humanising' of cow's milk is to increase the sugar content. This is done either by adding more lactose or other sugars like sucrose, fructose, glucose and dextri-maltose. Except for the colonisation of the gut by the potentially dangerous *E. coli* instead of the normal *Lactobacillus*, no immediate ill-effects have been reported as a result of feeding these abnormal sugars in early life. However, long-term ill-effects cannot be ruled out. For example, an association between inflammatory bowel disease and ingestion of refined sugars has been reported in adults. Also, endocrine responses in bottle-fed infants are significantly different from those who are breast-fed. The contrived and synthetic nature of many infant formulae together with the presence of 'unnatural' carbohydrates may play a role in setting the metabolism of formula-fed infants at a different level.

HUMAN MILK AS A NUTRIENT

In each mammalian species, the milk has evolved together with the mammal to provide the offspring with nutrition best adapted to the environment. Thus, in the whale the milk contains large amounts of fat to help the infant lay down body fat for protection against cold and to aid buoyancy. In the kangaroo, the mother has two separate nipples, each producing milk of different compositions. The new-born kangaroo is first attached to one nipple, where he obtains milk of high protein concentration. When the offspring is grown and can leave the pouch for brief periods, he changes over to the other nipple and obtains from it milk of different composition.

The attempts of the food chemist to modify the milk of one mammal, the cow, for feeding another, the human infant, have been largely unsuccessful, notwithstanding the claims made in the promotional literature. The reasons are obvious. It is not just the question of adding a sugar to get the carbohydrate content right, or of diluting to get the protein content right, nor of replacing butter fat with a mixture of vegetable oils. The entire structure of the protein in human milk is so very different from that in cow's milk (figure 4.1). The fatty acid

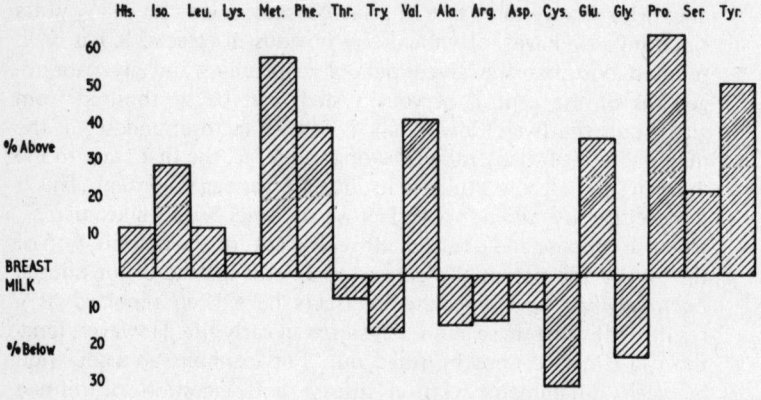

Figure 4.1 Comparison of the amino acid pattern of human and cow's milk protein using human milk protein as the standard. (The values, expressed as mg amino acid per g nitrogen in cow's milk, have been calculated as a percentage of those for breast milk expressed on the same basis.) (*Source:* Food and Agriculture Organization of the United Nations, 1970.)

composition is unique for each mother and so also are the electrolytes and trace elements. It is not surprising that the history of artificial feeding of infants is full of examples of one mishap after another – starting with rickets in the early part of the century, neonatal tetany in the early 1950s, pyridoxine deficiency in the late 1950s and 1960s and haemolysis due to vitamin E deficiency and risks of hypernatraemia (high blood sodium) in more recent years. Products promoted as 'ideal foods' are withdrawn a few years later when their shortcomings are discovered, only to be replaced by another family of products which are again promoted with equal vigour.

The uniqueness of the mother's milk in the nutrition of her infant is apparent when we consider the cellular mechanism of synthesis and secretion of its various constituents. Hormonal stimulation throughout pregnancy prepares the breasts for secretion of milk. Soon after the birth of the baby there is secretion of prolactin from the anterior pituitary. Together with other hormonal changes, it provides the stimulus for the activities of the several enzymes in the acinar cells of the mammary glands, leading to the synthesis and secretion of milk. Various cell organelles participate in the process. Synthesis occurs on the ribosomes in the rough endoplasmic reticulum in accordance with the genetic message carried within the cell nucleus. Thus, whereas the ribosomes and the rough endoplasmic reticulum provide the framework for the site of synthesis, the biological characteristics of the final product are determined by the DNA and the mRNA operating from the cell nucleus. The Golgi apparatus provides storage for the final product until it is emptied into the cell lumen (figure 4.2). The raw materials for milk synthesis

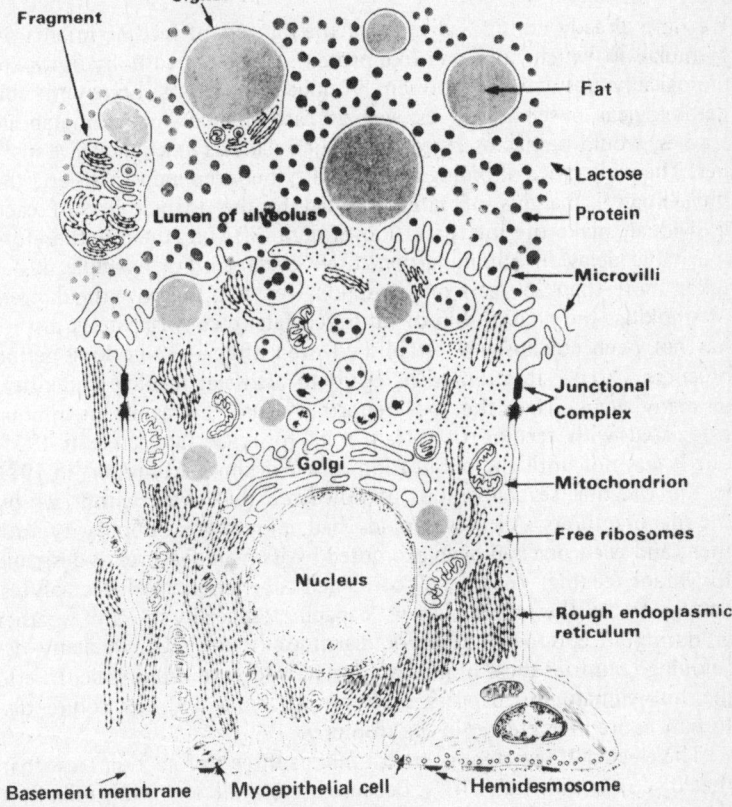

Figure 4.2   Ultrastructure of the secretory cell

come from the mother's body either as substances circulating in the blood, e.g. amino acids, or as products stored in her tissues, e.g. fats. Ultimately they are all derived from her diet. Thus, the interaction of the genetic constitution of the mother with her environment provides the raw material for the synthesis of milk in ways determined by the genetic code in the nucleus of the alveolar cell. The infant, on the other hand, is endowed by the mother with half of his genetic make-up. Hence from the biological point of view mother's milk is most suited for the unique metabolic activity of the infant's tissues. No amount of dilution, addition, adjusting or so-called humanising of the milk of another mammal will give the characteristic configuration of molecules and biological properties of a mother's milk for her offspring.

DANGERS OF ARTIFICIAL FEEDING

We have already considered some of the dangers of feeding infants on formulae in which nutrients like proteins, fats, and carbohydrates are biologically unsuitable or present in unusual amounts. Long-term epidemiological observations, as well as carefully conducted metabolic studies, would be necessary to prove such dangers in a conclusive manner. The wide range of biological variability between individuals and the physiological margins of safety, added to the adaptability of each individual, make the interpretation of data difficult; there is therefore inevitable delay in obtaining conclusive evidence. For example, it has taken more than 25 years of painstaking research to prove the dangers of smoking; the relationship of saturated fats to coronary heart disease has not been conclusively established even after a similar long period of enquiry. The situation with regard to artificial feeding is identical in many ways. Thus the first reports of hypernatraemia in infants, associated with feeding of certain milk formulae, appeared in 1955, but it was not until the publication of a Working Party report in 1974 in the UK that several brands of powdered milk were withdrawn by the manufacturers. All these brands had enjoyed great popularity until then, and each one had been promoted by its manufacturer as desirable for infant feeding. Yet they all contained large amounts of electrolytes, enough to tax the infant kidneys' capacity, especially in warm weather or during an episode of fever or diarrhoea (figure 4.3). In many developing countries these brands of milk powders are still on sale. Due to the hot climate the dangers of hypernatraemia and electrolyte disturbances are even greater in the tropics.

The electrolyte content of breast milk is three to four times less than that of cow's milk (table 4.7). Because breast milk and cow's milk have the same calorie content per given volume, infants fed cow's milk will

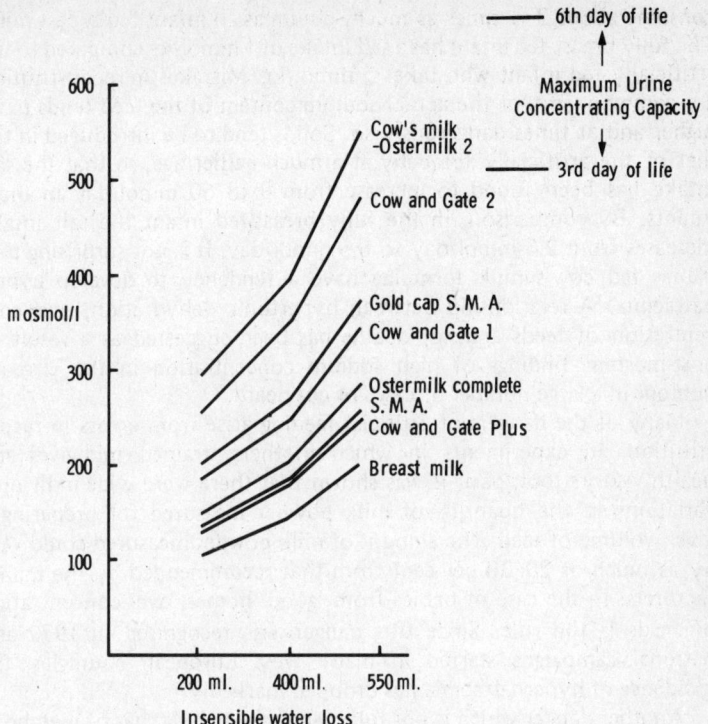

Figure 4.3 Urine osmolar load in a 5kg infant fed different milk formulae at 200ml/kg/day with varying insensible loss

Table 4.7 *The electrolyte and mineral content of human and cow's milk (m mol/litre)*

	Na	K	Cl	Ca	Mg	P
Human milk mean	6.5	15.4	12.1	8.8	1.2	4.8
(range)	(4.8–8.7)	(14.6–15.9)	(9.9–15.5)	(8.0–9.0)	(1.1–1.3)	(4.5–4.8)
Cow's milk mean	21.7	38.5	26.8	30.0	5.0	30.6
(range)	(15.2–39.1)	(28.2–43.6)	(25.4–31.0)	(27.5–32.5)	(3.8–5.8)	(29.0–32.3)

Source: DHSS (1977) and (1980).

consume about 3-4 times as much sodium as an infant fed breast milk. The fully breast-fed infant has a salt intake of 1 mmol/kg compared to the artificially fed infant who takes 5 mmol/kg. Mistakes in reconstitution are common, so that the actual sodium content of the feed tends to be higher and at times dangerously so. Solids tend to be introduced in the diet of the artificially fed baby at a much earlier age, so that the salt intake has been found to increase from 9 to 60 mmol/day in these infants. By comparison, in the fully breast-fed infant the salt intake increases from 2.6 mmol/day to 6.5 mmol/day. It is not surprising that babies fed cow's milk formulae have a tendency to develop hypernatraemia. A relationship between hypertonic dehydration, over-concentration of feeds and cot deaths has been suggested as a result of post-mortem findings of high sodium concentration in the vitreous humour in a large number of cases of cot death.

Many of the dangers of artificial feeding arise from errors in reconstitution. In experiments in which mothers, trained midwives and health visitors took part, it was shown that there were wide individual variations in the quantity of milk powder measured for preparing a given volume of feed. The amount of milk powder measured could vary by as much as 20-30 per cent from that recommended by the manufacturers. In the case of babies from 'good' homes, over-concentration of feeds is the rule. Since this danger was recognised in 1972 and national campaigns started in many West European countries, the incidence of hypernatraemia has dropped markedly.

Another danger which is not fully recognised yet is that of metabolic acidosis. Most infant formulae which are based on cow's milk present a greater acid load to the infant compared to breast milk. There is a significantly higher likelihood of acidosis in bottle-fed infants. Diarrhoea and dehydration in bottle-fed infants carry the added risk of metabolic acidosis besides hypernatraemia. As with the solute load, the pH falls with concentration of feeds, each extra scoop lowering the pH by 0.05 in the case of some brands.

The dangers of artificial feeding are most obvious in Third World countries. Breast feeding has declined sharply in these countries in the face of intensive promotion by the manufacturers, and in the absence of a strong professional and governmental support for breast feeding. Many mothers take to artificial feeding only to find that the family income is inadequate to pay for the cost of powdered milk. In one survey of ten countries in the Third World it was revealed that the cost of artificial feeding a 6 month-old infant could be as much as a third to a half of the minimum wage. In fact, because of the high levels of unemployment, many wage-earners accept employment at wages far lower than the statutory minimum wage. Thus the true cost of artificial feeding could well be a sizeable proportion of the family income. The temptation to 'stretch' the tin of milk powder is only too great in such a situation, with consequent underfeeding of the infant. In 1972, in Barbados, only 18 per cent of the poorer mothers were using a 1lb (0.45 kg) tin of powdered milk for 4 days or less, as indicated by the manufacturer. The majority extended the use of the milk from 5 days to as much as 3 weeks. It is not surprising, therefore, that the decline of breast feeding in the developing world is accompanied by a high incidence of undernutrition in children. An additional danger in the overcrowded homes of the poor is that of infected feeds due to lack of hygiene and the inability to care for the feeding bottles and mixing utensils properly. Diarrhoeal illness in early infancy and in the absence of adequate primary health care facilities can be life-threatening. It has been estimated by UNICEF that every year 1 million infant deaths occur in the world due to causes related to bottle-feeding, directly or indirectly. The survivors of the initial episode of diarrhoea often face a vicious cycle of malnutrition and recurrent diarrhoea, often terminating in death due to diarrhoea or malnutrition. The long-term effects of inflammatory bowel disease so early in life need further study. It has been postulated that chronic inflammatory bowel diseases like Crohn's disease and ulcerative colitis may have their beginnings in infective diarrhoea of early infancy.

HUMAN MILK AS A PROTECTIVE AGENT

Mother's milk is not only a source of nourishment for the baby, but also a powerful antimicrobial agent. Breast milk contains several factors which act in concert to form a biological system for protection against infection. For a long time epidemiological evidence has been indicating the benefits of breast feeding as regards protection from infection. When 1712 mothers in rural Chile were interviewed to assess the effect of feeding practices on the health of infants, it was found that if bottle-feeding commenced before the age of 3 months, the mortality was three times that in breast-fed babies. Similarly, in the study of patterns of mortality in childhood conducted by the Pan American Health Organisation in South America in 1973, it was found that breast feeding was a major factor in infant survival. More recently epidemiological studies have revealed the protective effect of breast feeding against a variety of viruses including the respiratory syncytial virus.

In the early days almost half the protein in breast milk is in an immunologically active form either as lactoferrin or as one of the immunoglobulins or as complement (table 4.8). Even though the concentration of IgA and lactoferrin declines as lactation proceeds, the immunologi-

Table 4.8 *Immunologically active proteins of human milk (mg/100 ml)*

	Day 5	Days 8-28	Days 50-200
Immunoglobulin A	490	151	148
Immunoglobulin M	12	4	1
Immunoglobulin G	32	32	1
Complement (C_3 and C_4)	7	2.5	1.5
Lysozyme	10	10	10
Lactoferrin	550	300	150
α-antitrypsin	10	5	–
Total (mg/100 ml)	1111	504.5	311.5
Total protein (g/100 ml)	2	2	1.5
Total volume of milk (ml/24 hours)	500	750	900-1000

Source: McClelland, D. B. L., McGrath, J. and Samson, R. R. *Acta Paed. Scand.* (1978), Suppl. 271.

cally active proteins still constitute a large proportion of the total protein of breast milk.

The various protective factors in breast milk and their modes of action are described below.

Immunoglobulins (Figure 4.4(a) and 4.4(b))

Breast milk contains IgA, IgM, IgG and IgD. Of these, IgA occurs in the largest amounts and has been shown to play an important biological role. The concentration of IgA in breast milk is higher than in the mother's serum, indicating active secretion rather than passive transfer. Also, it is present as a dimer, whereas in the serum it occurs as a monomer. The two molecules of the dimer are joined together by a polypeptide chain called the J chain. The composite molecule is more resistant than serum IgA to pH changes and enzymic attacks and is therefore active in the infant's gut. In several studies the antibodies carried in the IgA of the milk have been demonstrated in the stools of the breast-fed infant in amounts directly proportional to the intake of milk.

The IgG in breast milk also serves an important anti-infection function. It is known that during pregnancy IgG passes from the mother's blood to the infant through the placenta. Early studies on human colo-

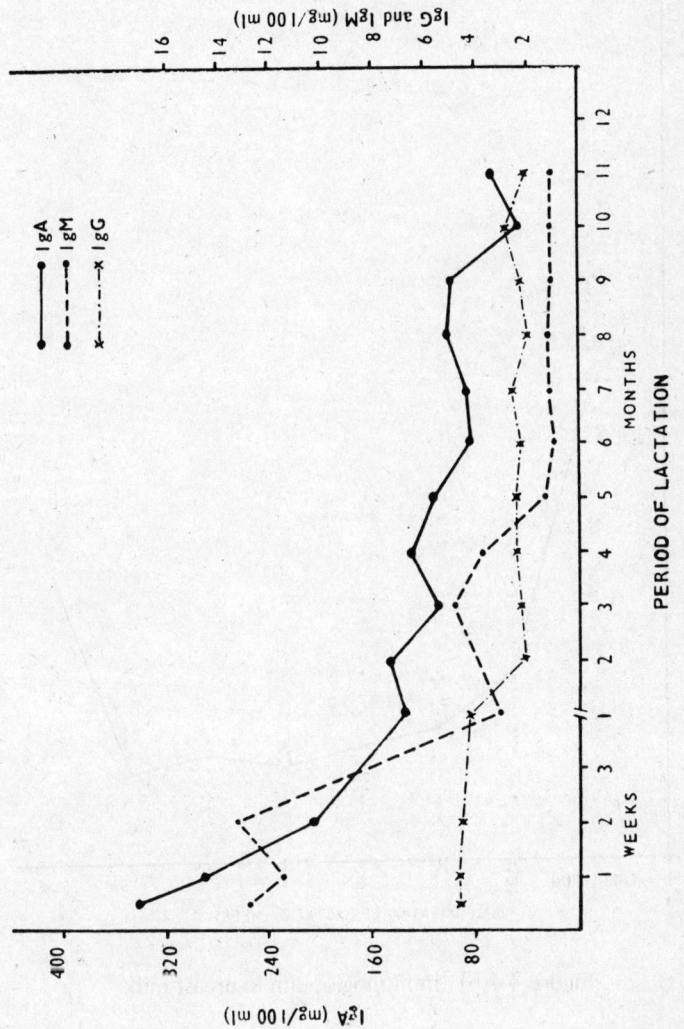

Figure 4.4(a) Immunoglobulins in breast milk

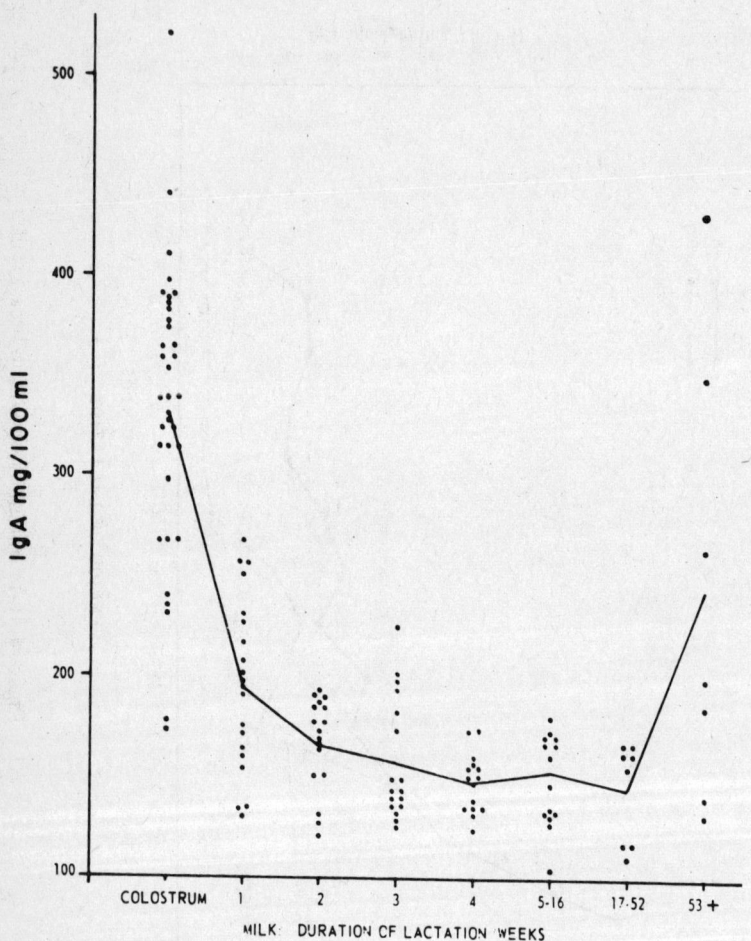

Figure 4.4(b) Immunoglobulin in breast milk

strum did not show the presence of *large* amounts of IgG and it was thought that in the case of the human the only mechanism of transfer was through the placenta. However, breast-fed babies have higher levels of serum IgG at 4-6 weeks compared to bottle-fed controls. Since the baby receives a considerable amount of IgG transplacentally, there is presumably no urgency for large quantities to be provided through the colostrum after birth, as is the case with the calf and the pig. Instead, the breast-fed human infant receives IgG in small doses over a prolonged period.

Antibodies

Breast milk contains antibodies against many organisms, both viral and bacterial. Most of these antibodies are of the IgA type and a large proportion of them are directed against *E. coli*, though antibodies against tetanus, *Shigella*, *Haemophilus pertussis*, *Vibrio cholerae* and *V. pneumoniae* have also been demonstrated.

There is experimental evidence to show that *E. coli* antibody in breast milk is specific against the *E. coli* in the mother's gut. In one experiment, pregnant women were administered *E. coli* of an unusual nature, and it was found that even though there was no *serum* antibody response, breast milk contained antibodies against the same *E. coli*. It would thus appear that plasma cells in the gut wall of the mother become sensitised to bacterial antigens in the gut lumen, and then move through the blood stream to 'home in' on the mammary gland where they contribute the specific antibody to the milk.

Lactoferrin (Figure 4.5)

An iron-binding protein in breast milk, lactoferrin, plays a key role in the action of IgA on the bacterium *E. coli* by inhibiting the proliferation of this organism in the gut of the newborn. Breast milk contains large quantities of lactoferrin, 2-6 mg/ml. It has a high affinity for ferric iron which *E. coli* require for growth and multiplication. Lactoferrin thus deprives *E. coli* of iron and bacterial proliferation is slowed. In laboratory experiments it can be demonstrated that In the presence of lactoferrin only traces of antibody are required to produce bacteriostasis. When excess iron is added, the lactoferrin is saturated and its action against *E. coli* is lost.

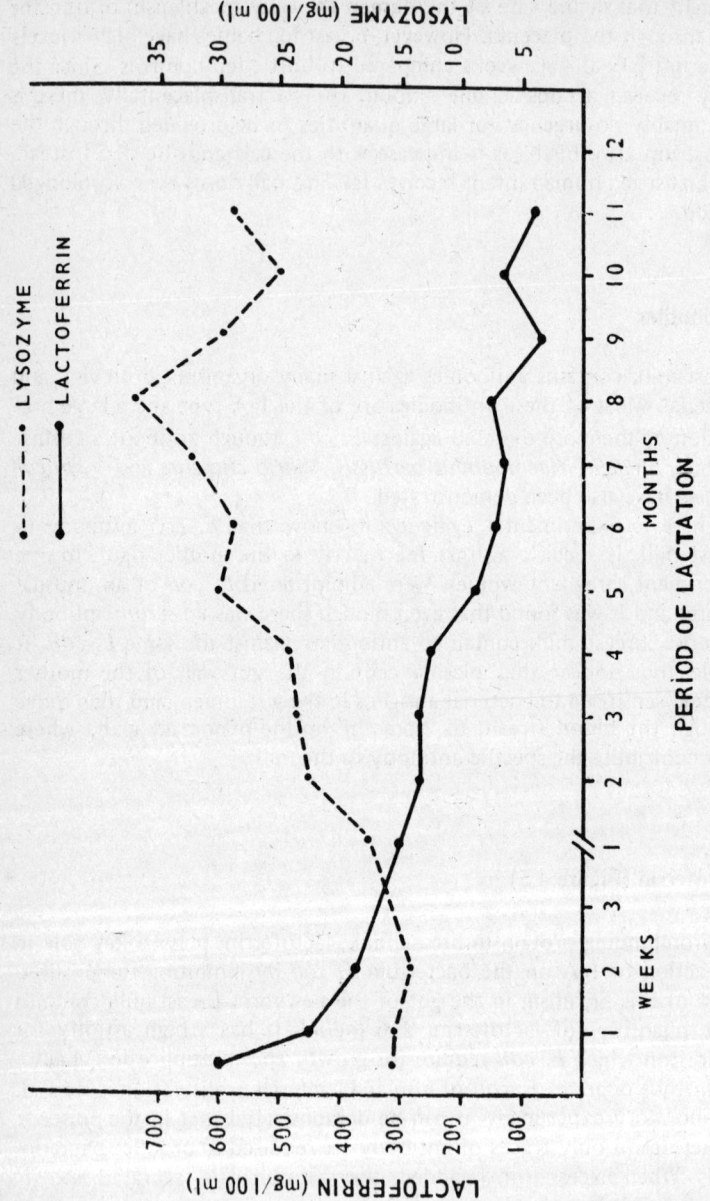

Figure 4.5 Lactoferrin and lysozome in breast milk

Lymphocytes and macrophages

Human milk contains a large number of cells varying from 2000 to 4000 cells/mm^3. These are of two main types: the lymphocyte and the macrophage. The lymphocytes are immunologically active and synthesise IgA as well as β1c complement. They are the type of cells which 'home in' on the mammary gland after being sensitised to bacterial antigens in the mother's gut, and they secrete specific antibodies against these bacteria. The macrophages of breast milk are capable of destroying *Klebsiella*, *Staphylococcus aureus* and *E. coli in vitro* after opsonisation by the aqueous phase of milk. The efficiency with which these organisms are killed is as good as that in the case of blood leucocytes in serum. In addition, the macrophages and neutrophils from human milk can be shown to phagocytose *Candida albicans*. In animal models which were appropriately stressed by hypoxia they were also shown to protect against necrotising enterocolitis.

Animal studies indicate that the cells in breast milk may have a role to play beyond the lumen of the gut. Transfer of tuberculin sensitivity demonstrated in the case of the human infant is an example of such a role. It would appear that besides being immunologically active in the gastrointestinal tract the 'live' components of breast milk act as transmitters of immunologic information and help prepare the immune system of the newborn for meeting environmental challenges. For example, a substantial increase in the secretory IgA content of nasal and salivary mucus has been found in breast-fed infants as compared to those who are bottle-fed during the early neonatal period. It has been suggested that this may be due to a soluble cell factor in milk activating the developing immune mechanisms of the infant. The presence of such an immunoregulatory factor has been confirmed in laboratory experiments using colostral cells.

Other factors

Breast milk contains large amounts of the C_3 and C_4 components of complement, which can be activated in experimental conditions by the antibody contained in the IgA of the milk. It also contains lysozyme in large amounts. The exact mechanism of action of these substances has not yet been fully determined. It has been postulated that they interact together as a biological system in mounting immunological attacks on bacteria in the baby's gut.

In addition there is the bifidus factor which promotes the growth of the *Lactobacillus* organism under the specific pH and chemical environment of the neonatal gut generated by breast milk. The gut flora of the artificially fed infant is made up largely of *E. coli*, with some *Streptococcus faecalis*, in contrast to the breast-fed infant in whom the lactobacillus predominates. The *E. coli* harboured by the gut of the artificially fed infant constitute a reservoir of potential pathogens. The exact conditions under which they can cause disease are not yet understood. The immune factors in breast milk will keep the number of *E. coli* in the gut low until such time as the baby has developed his own immunity. In this way breast milk is unique. It is an agent which protects at the same time as it nourishes and the mammary gland performs a function not very different from that of the placenta in intrauterine life.

Closely related to protection from infection is the role of human milk in preventing hypersensitivity. Secretory IgA in the gut lumen is known to prevent the adsorption of antigen onto the gut mucosa. When there is a deficiency of IgA, macromolecules of antigen in the gut lumen are able to pass through the mucosal cells and enter the blood stream or lymphatics and trigger an immune response. Breast milk, with its high content of IgA, prevents the escape of antigen into the blood stream and thus protects against atopic disease.

Recently it has been shown that breast milk contains a rich variety of substances, the significance of which has not yet been fully understood. It contains small amounts of several hormones like corticosteroids, prolactin, thyrotrophin and thyroxine. It also contains biological mediators of hormone function in the form of cyclic nucleotides, *viz*. cyclic AMP and cyclic GMP. Both the latter substances are known to participate in the regulation of proliferation and differentiation processes associated with the growth and maturation of the newborn. Studies in rats have shown that the stomach content of both these cyclic nucleotides remained high for at least 1 hour after a feed, indicating their availability for absorption in the gut.

BIOLOGICAL MEDIATOR: A NEW ROLE FOR BREAST MILK

The hormonal responses to feeding are different between breast-fed and bottle-fed infants. Blood levels of insulin and of gut hormones like motilin, enteroglucagon, neurotensin and pancreatic polypeptide show significant changes following a feed in bottle-fed infants. In the case of breast-fed infants these changes are much reduced or absent. Basal levels of the hormones also tend to be higher in bottle-fed infants. Since some of these hormones are likely to play a key role in neonatal adaptation, only future research can demonstrate the long-term benefits of breast-feeding. However, when one considers the properties of human breast milk in the fields of nutrition, immunology, endocrinology and developmental biology, a new biological role of breast milk becomes obvious. It is not merely a nutritious broth to be compared with processed products marketed in cans or ready-to-feed bottles. It is a biological mediator carrying a rich variety of substances which can trigger and control extrauterine adaptation of the infant for intact and healthy survival.

MOTHER-INFANT RELATIONSHIP

The act of suckling is a form of intimate communication between the mother and her infant, and it contributes to the creation of the love bond between the two. The skin contact, the eye-to-eye or 'en face' position adopted during or soon after feeding, the satisfaction of hunger in the infant and the pleasurable tactile stimulation in the mother during suckling all promote, as well as add to, the process of bonding between the two. In many mammals, the time of birth is a critical period during which imprinting occurs, so that the mother recognises her offspring and vice-versa. Similar imprinting during a critical post-partum period also occurs in the human, and breast feeding plays an important role in this process. Mothers who are separated from their infants, for medical or other reasons, at this critical period, have a higher incidence of rejection of their babies and of child abuse.

THE SPACING OF PREGNANCIES

It is estimated that more conceptions are prevented through lactational amenorrhoea than all the contraceptive methods put together. Certainly in the rural areas of the developing world breast feeding and abstinence are the only two practical methods of contraception which are universally available. Rural studies in Nigeria, Senegal, Rwanda, Bangladesh and Java showed a postponement of menstruation by more than a year in breast feeding women compared with those who did not breast feed. In Korea, Taiwan and India, a postponement of between 8 and 12 months has been found. By comparison, women who do not breast feed return to regular menstruation in about 3 months after the birth of the baby.

The contraceptive effect of breast feeding is due to the surges of prolactin in the mother's blood which occur as reflex responses to the tactile stimulation of the nipple during suckling. Prolactin in turn has an inhibitory effect on ovarian activity. The contraceptive effect is therefore maximum when breast feeding is on demand, complete and unrestricted both during the day as well as the night. The contraceptive effect is greatly reduced if breast feeding is partial and supplemented early with solids or cow's milk formulae. By prolonging the birth interval on-demand breast feeding ensures adequate mothering of the infant, which is yet another way in which it contributes to the protection of the infant.

INTERVENTION PROGRAMMES

The data presented in the foregoing pages help to establish breast milk as an important biological agent for the survival and extrauterine adaptation of the newborn. In all societies morbidity and mortality rates are higher in artificially fed infants compared to those who are fully breast-fed. Studies in Europe and the United States at the beginning of the century showed that mortality rates were 3 to 6 times higher in artificially fed infants. Even as recently as the 1940s the mortality risk for artificially fed infants was 2 to 3 times that for breast-fed infants *in all social groups* in Sweden. It was only from the 1940s onwards that reports from industrialised countries began to suggest equal mortality rates for both groups of infants. This is not so much due to the availability of improved products as to improved environmental hygiene. In the developing world, where more than three-quarters of the world's babies are born, the mortality risks continue to be high. It can be stated without reservation that if in the rural area of a developing country an infant has no access to the mother's milk, then the chances of survival will be very slim indeed. The greatest danger is from progressive undernutrition resulting in marasmus, and from diarrhoeal disease. The decline in breast feeding in the developing world has been associated with a rise in the incidence of marasmus and diarrhoea, especially amongst the urban poor.

Alarmed at the hazards of bottle feeding, the international agencies have been voicing concern since 1970 at the high-pressure advertising of baby foods in the developing world. Finally in 1981 the 34th World Health Assembly voted (with one dissenting vote) in favour of an international code of ethics for member states to adopt in their countries.

From the outset three major factors have been identified as contributing to the marked and rapid decline in breast feeding. These are the promotional practices of baby-food manufacturers and the absence of a unified and strong stand by the health profession against such promotion and in favour of breast feeding. Thirdly, and most surprisingly, governments of the Third World have hitherto failed to look upon breast milk as an important national resource, despite the large expenditure in foreign exchange on the importation of various brands of powdered milk.

Even though the health profession has an important and active role to play for the protection of breast feeding, there is need for support at the community and national level. The specific interventions should therefore be considered at the level of the health profession, the community and the nation.

Health profession-related interventions

(1) In all training institutions there should be adequate time allowed to teaching about breast feeding, including its practical management. The clinical, nutritional, public health and social benefits of breast feeding need to be emphasised together with the harmful effects of bottle feeding.
(2) Present-day medical practices, proven to be obstacles to successful breast feeding, need to be modified (table 4.9).
(3) A generally positive attitude towards breast feeding in hospital wards and clinics will encourage mothers to breast feed. For example, mothers who have successfully breast fed their infants may be utilised as 'counsellors' and 'demonstrators' in the antenatal and under-5s clinics. Small discussion groups of first-time lactating mothers may be set up in under-5s clinics utilising such counsellors to discuss problems and their management. A rational policy for hospital admission of children so that breast feeding mothers are admitted with their sick children, and 'lodger babies' are admitted with their sick mothers will also help create a generally positive attitude towards breast feeding. Most important, of course, are the policies and routines of the maternity wards. Simple modifications of hospital routines such as, for example, more relaxed attitude towards visiting by the husband and family in the maternity wards, rooming-in, permissive feeding schedules for babies and so on have been known to raise the incidence of breast feeding. There are also other benefits like *reduced* incidence of neonatal sepsis and improved survival rates of low birth weight babies.
(4) Besides a generally supportive attitude towards breast feeding in everyday medical practice, professional bodies also need to be active in the community and nationally to advocate breast feeding. In countries where medical and nursing associations have repeatedly advocated breast feeding, national policies and supportive legislation have eventually emerged. In this respect it is necessary to join hands with community and national groups like the local branches of La Leche League and the Consumers' Association.

Table 4.9 *Practices interfering with successful lactation*

Practices	Effect on lactation	Modifications
Delaying first breast feed.	Inadequate stimulation of let-down reflex.	Putting infant to the breast immediately after birth.
Excess maternal anaesthesia resulting in sedated newborn.	Weak, unco-ordinated suckling.	Avoidance of excessive sedation of the mother.
Supplying prelacteal glucose feeds.	Weakening of the stimulus.	Avoidance.
The rigid 4-hourly routine of feeding with no night feeds.	Confused mother resulting in anxiety, and a hungry fretful baby.	Frequent on-demand feeding during the day as well as the night.
Separation of the infant from the mother.	Suppression of lactation.	Rooming-in.
Uninformed, unsupported mother.	Interference with the let-down reflex.	Preparation of the mother for lactation during pregnancy and counselling from lactation 'advisers' with emotional support in puerperium.
Excessive use of instrumental delivery (pain + anaesthesia)	Suppression of lactation.	Avoidance.
Unsympathetic, inexperienced staff.	Anxiety and frustration in the mother.	Adequately trained staff skilled in the management of breast feeding.
Provision of 'gift packs', visits by 'milk nurses' and use of posters and brochures advertising baby foods.	Suppression of let-down reflex and drying-up of milk, e.g. by the trial of the gift pack.	Hospital policies prohibiting all such practices.

INTERVENTIONS AT THE COMMUNITY LEVEL

The importance of community groups like the La Leche League and Consumers' Associations in reversing the trend from bottle feeding has been well documented in Western Europe and North America. Besides being supportive of local mothers who are breast feeding, such groups also help to collate and exchange information nationally as well as internationally. Such community groups can also act as 'watchdog' bodies monitoring the promotional practices of the baby-food manufacturers.

INTERVENTIONS AT THE NATIONAL LEVEL

Community pressure groups and national professional bodies can often succeed in persuading governments to formulate national strategies of mother and child welfare. Many governments now recognise the unique role of the mother in national development through raising the citizens of tomorrow. In addition, the concepts of human breast milk as a national resource, and the wastage in foreign exchange if breast feeding is allowed to decline, are now fully appreciated by most national planners. The most effective step for any government to take is to enforce the ethical code suggested by the World Health Organisation with regard to the promotion of infant feeding formulae. To confuse the issue the infant-food industry has come up with meaningless codes and has persuaded some countries to adopt them. Good examples of forceful national legislations are those of Burma and Papua-New Guinea where the sale of formulae and feeding bottles is prohibited except on prescription. The legislation also prohibits advertising in the mass media. In Mozambique, besides control of advertisements, free importation of a variety of brands of powdered milk has been stopped. Instead the government imports the 'best-buy' brand and distributes it through the health service with a national label.

As more women enter the labour force, there will be a growing need for a variety of facilities to enable the working mother to breast feed her baby. Many such facilities may need to be backed by appropriate legislation. Thus, adequate and paid maternity leave, creches near the work-places, nursing breaks during the work day and flexi-hours for the working mother are all examples of ways in which a society can acknowledge the unique contribution of the working mother to the national economy.

FURTHER READING

Ebrahim, G. J. *Breast Feeding - the biological option.* Macmillan, Basingstoke and London, 1978.
Jelliffe, D. B. and Jelliffe, E. F. P. *Human Milk in the Modern World.* Oxford University Press, Oxford, New York and Toronto, 1978.

World Health Organization. *Contemporary Patterns of Breast Feeding.* Report on the WHO Collaborative Study on Breast Feeding. World Health Organization, Geneva, 1981.

World Health Organization. *Breastfeeding. A brochure for ready reference.* WHO, Geneva (n.d.).

Chapter 5

The Weaning Period

Most infants thrive well on their mother's milk alone in the first 3-4 months of life. This is a period of rapid growth. The average infant is expected to increase his birth weight by more than half and grow in length by 10 per cent during this time. The demands for nutrients are higher than at any time in life. It is estimated that the normal 2-3 month-old infant is likely to consume 116 kcal/kg/day and probably absorbs more than 100 kcal/kg/day. By contrast a 70 kg young adult male will rarely absorb as much as 50 kcal/kg/day. Thus the infant's digestive tract is more remarkable for its high capacity for absorption than for any limitations; it is functioning close to capacity in order to keep up with the demands of rapid growth. Approximately one-third of the energy intake between birth and the age of 4 months may be accounted for by synthesis of new tissues. By contrast, during the growth spurt of puberty, which is another period of rapid growth, the adolescent utilises less than 10 per cent of his energy intake for growth, even during periods of peak growth.

At various times doubts have been expressed about the ability of breast milk to satisfy the nutritional needs of pre-term and small-for-date (SFD) infants, as well as of older, healthy infants, especially in developing countries. Recent studies have demonstrated a greater concentration of protein in the milk of mothers delivering pre-term infants. The mean concentrations of protein, sodium, chloride and potassium in early pre-term milk have been found to be adequate to meet the estimated requirements for the pre-term infant (table 5.1).

Nutrient balance studies show that on their mothers' milk, pre-term infants retain nitrogen at the same rate as during the period of intrauterine growth. Fat absorption by pre-term infants is superior on breast milk compared to any other type of feeding. So also is the protein and amino-acid status. Moreover metabolic difficulties like raised blood levels of amino acids, acidosis, and high blood urea do not arise. The greatest advantage, especially for developing countries, and outweighing every other consideration, is the immunological protection provided by

Table 5.1 Composition of milk in mothers delivering pre-term infants

	Pre-term delivery	Full-term delivery
Nitrogen (mg/dl)	328	196
Fat (g/dl)	3.80	3.75
Lactose (g/dl)	5.23	6.50
Calories (kcal/dl)	70	67

Source: Atkinson, S. A. et al. J. Paed. (1981), 99, 618.

the mother's milk. Several control studies from different parts of the world are now available all showing a lower incidence of sepsis in these high-risk infants when they are fed their mothers' milk.

The greatest anxiety at present is about the SFD infant. A large proportion of such infants reflect varying periods of malnutrition in fetal life. The several contributory factors including lack of adequate care in pregnancy have been discussed in Chapter 3. Two additional factors also need to be taken into account. In the case of a large majority of such mothers, weight gain during pregnancy is less than normal, indicating inadequate body stores in the mother. Secondly, breast milk output has been shown to be related to the size of the infant. In general, mothers with smaller babies produce less milk than those with larger infants. The reason is not known and further studies are necessary. It is likely that the combination of factors which limit fetal growth also limit the lactational performance of the mother. Here, seasonal factors are also important. In the rural society, the wet season is the most stressful period for subsistence farmers. As described earlier this is the time of the 'hungry months', high demands for physical work and high prevalence of illness, especially malaria and diarrhoea. Depending upon the time of the year when a baby was conceived, and the work load of the mother, the stresses of the wet season may be severe enough to affect fetal growth. Similarly, heavy seasonal work causing reduction in the milk output of the mother will have more serious effect in the first 4-6 months of life of the infant. Finally, the whole question of maternal malnutrition, heavy physical work, and inadequate fetal growth is associated with the problem of poverty. It is amongst the rural and urban poor that the incidence of low birth weight is high and hence the need for health and nutrition care the greatest. Under these circumstances the immunological properties of breast milk make it the most important vehicle for the protection of the SFD infant. Several studies indicate that such infants have low levels of cell-mediated immunity, persisting for several years. Hence the immunological safeguards provided by breast milk are all the more necessary for such infants. The need therefore is for continuation of breast feeding into the second year of life and even longer.

Lastly, the question of adequacy of breast milk as the sole nutrient for the older infant in developing countries. It has been suggested that after the third month of life the output of breast milk is not enough to meet the energy and protein requirements of the growing infant. Such considerations must obviously depend on reliable data on the energy and nutrient requirements of the infant at different ages, as well as the accuracy of measurement of the milk output. Calculations of the energy and nutrient requirement recommended by FAO/WHO (1973) are based on the intakes of 142 normally growing bottle-fed babies in North America. These requirements would be supplied by a breast milk output of 850 ml/day. Many would agree that a milk output of 750–800 ml/day at 2–4 months is more typical of well-nourished mothers in affluent societies.

Milk output is usually measured by test-weighing the infant. Here too there are obvious pitfalls like, for example, the suppression of the let-down reflex by the various interferences necessary for the procedure. Added to this is the practical impossibility of weighing the infant after every single feed in communities where frequent on-demand feeding is the general rule. Lastly, more recent work, with feeding infants known quantities of milk by the bottle and test-weighing afterwards, has shown that the scientific validity of test-weighing as a reliable method is doubtful.

The WHO collaborative study conducted in nine countries and involving 22 857 mother/infant pairs showed that the growth of children, including those in the lower income groups, tended to be satisfactory up to the age of 6 months by the WHO reference standards. The physical evidence of adequate growth is more convincing than theoretical calculations based on requirements and milk outputs as assessed by test-weighing. However, the cautionary message of the latter studies is important, and there is a need for optimising milk output in nursing mothers by attending to their nutrition and encouraging repeated on-demand feeding in preference to schedules adapted from bottle-feeding regimes.

It is remarkable that breast milk alone can supply all the nutrients necessary to support rapid growth in early infancy. Studies on growth of infants in the Gambia, Uganda and Guatemala have shown that in many instances the rate of growth may even be greater than that of English or American infants of the same age. The output of breast milk keeps pace with demand until about the age of 3–4 months, and at times even longer, when it reaches the maximum and cannot increase further. It is at this time that the growth of a large proportion of children in the developing world begins to slow down. Thus in Uganda it was found that there is a sharp fall in the velocity of weight gain between the ages of 3 and 6 months, and a further fall between 6 and 9 months to a rate of only half of that in English children. After the age of 9 months the velocity of weight gain gradually improves, but continues to be lower than that of English children until the age of 18 months. The rates of weight gain in the second and third years of life are similar to those of English children, but the ground lost in the early period is never made up. Growth in height also suffers in the same way. There is a sharp fall in the rate of increase in length from the age of 3 months, so that at 6 months the velocity of growth in height is less than 85 per cent of that of English children. It begins to improve at the age of 1 year and reaches the normal rate at about 1½ years, after which it continues at the normal rate in the second and third years. Again, the ground lost in the early period is not recovered. Thus growth in both weight and height is most severely affected between 3 and 12 months of age, and the slowing of growth in the first year of life accounts for 91 per cent of the deficit in body weight and 98 per cent of the deficit in length at the age of 3 years. Such a faltering of growth in the latter half of the first year of life is characteristic of the majority of children in the Third World. Though their rate of growth approaches the standard in the second and third years, when growth is normally slowing down, the lost ground is never recovered and the deficit remains.

DANGERS OF THE WEANING PERIOD

The weaning period is fraught with danger for a large proportion of the world's children and nutritional disorders are common at this time of life. In the West a general awareness of the nutritional needs of the weanling, together with the ability of the average family to provide the necessary foods, have helped to remove most of the dangers of the weaning period. In the peasant society, however, parents are generally unaware of the dietary needs of children, and several customs associated with weaning are likely to give rise to nutritional deficiencies. For example, in many parts of India the ceremony of 'Anna Prasanna' must be carried out at the time of weaning. In this ceremony, several kinds of foods are cooked and offered to the deity to invoke her blessings. Family and kinsmen are entertained during the celebrations. Often weaning is delayed until such time as the family have been able to save for the expense of the ceremony. In Uganda and among several communities along the shores of Lake Victoria, the common practice is to separate the child from his mother in order to take him off the breast and to get him to eat other foods. The weanling is sent away to live with the grandparents for a few months. The unhappiness of separation is added to the nutritional upset caused by a sudden change from a highly nutritious food to a starchy gruel.

In the traditional society weaning is commonly abrupt and unplanned. Often it is brought about by the occurrence of another pregnancy in the mother. In many communities there are superstitions and beliefs concerning the effects of another pregnancy on the quality of breast milk. It is believed that the heat from the womb 'poisons' the milk in the breasts. Also that the baby in the womb is jealous of the older sibling on the breast. It is therefore considered urgent that the child should be taken off the breast immediately. In the ensuing hurry, there is hardly any time for the gradual introduction of solids to allow the child to get used to them. Instead, the breast is denied to him. The mother may apply potions to her nipples so that when the child takes the breast, their sharp bitter taste makes him give up suckling. The practice of separating the mother from the child is yet another way of effecting abrupt weaning.

By the age of 6 months, weaning has commenced in most children with small supplements prepared out of local foods. Commonly it is a gruel or pap made from the local staple. Here again, traditional practices, advice from the elders or family members, and the mother's own experience determines the type and consistency of the weaning diet (figure 5.1).

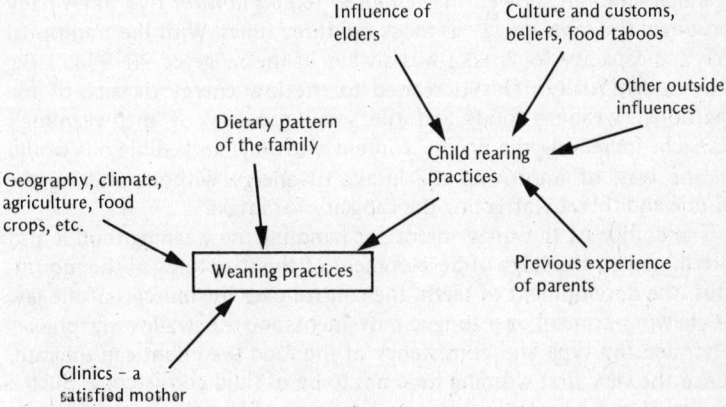

Figure 5.1. Determinants of weaning practices

TRADITIONAL DIETARY PRACTICES RESULTING IN LOW INTAKE OF ENERGY

In the traditional diet breast milk provides the foundations on to which other weaning foods can be gradually added. In a field study in Uganda it was noticed that during their second year breast-fed infants obtained 91 kcal/kg body weight and the non-breast-fed infants consumed 68 kcal/kg body weight per day. After breast feeding was stopped the intake of other foods was increased by 60 per cent, but it was still not sufficient to make up for the energy supplied by breast milk. The reason is that human breast milk has a relatively high energy density at 6 kcal/g dry matter and the transition to a diet of relatively low energy density is the cause of many nutritional problems. This concept of 'energy density' of the diet is an important advance in our knowledge of weaning foods.

Studies of food intake in young children from several countries confirm the above findings. In all peasant communities, energy intake with the traditional weaning foods is well below requirements. The intake of energy becomes inadequate soon after the third month and does not increase much between the ages of 7 and 30 months. Protein intake, though low, increases with age. The current view is that inadequate intake of energy, and not of protein, is the main aetiological factor in infantile malnutrition.

At first glance it may appear that the intake of energy could be increased by increasing the number of feeds offered to the child. In practice, however, this is not so simple. For example, the field study on Ugandan children showed that children fed *ad libitum* five times daily consumed the same energy as those fed three times. With the traditional diet, the capacity for intake was always in the range of 90–95 kcal/kg body weight daily. This is related to the low energy density of the traditional weaning foods and the small capacity of the weanling's stomach. Increasing the energy content with fats and edible oils would be one way of improving the intake of energy without altering the volume and thereby affecting the capacity for intake.

The ability of the small infant for handling the weaning food is also determined by the stage of development of the structures of the mouth. Thus, the development of teeth, the control over the muscles of the jaw for chewing, control over tongue movements and the swallowing reflexes determine the type and consistency of the food the infant can tolerate. Hence the very first weaning food has to be of fluid consistency. Such a thin gruel can have only very small content of the staple. Adding fats and oils to the gruel not only raises the energy content but also has the important effect of maintaining the gruel more fluid. At a given consistency a gruel cooked with oil can be made with more flour and less water and thereby the intake of other nutrients besides energy can be increased.

FOOD INTAKE AND APPETITE IN THE WEANLING

When daily food intakes in infants and young children are monitored over a period of time, the important role of appetite in the control of food intake becomes clear. In the study of Ugandan infants it was found that, below the age of 6 months, less than 10 per cent of children suffered from anorexia, but after that age lack of appetite was reported in 25-40 per cent by their mothers. The highest prevalence of poor appetite was in the age group between 13 and 18 months. Anorexia was often due to illness, the frequency of which rose sharply after the age of 6 months. The prevalence of anorexia can be appreciated from the fact that between the ages of 7 and 24 months, the average Ugandan child did not eat well on 1 day out of 3, and from the third year onwards 1 day out of 4.

Even when the child ate well, the traditional bulky food provided not more than 100 kcal/kg body weight daily. Such an intake is just enough for normal weight gain and for maintenance of serum albumin levels, but not for catch-up growth after an illness. If the energy density of the traditional food were to be raised from 100-125 kcal/100 g to 125-150 kcal/100 g by the means mentioned, the energy intake of a 10 kg child would be increased by 250 kcal/day. This increased energy intake will provide a small margin of safety for such periods when food intake is diminished by anorexia. Again, the importance of breast milk in the *second year* of life is well demonstrated by this study. By providing additional energy and protein it helps to offset the energy constraints of the traditional weaning foods. The mean daily intake of energy in infants who were not breast fed was barely adequate for maintenance even with a good appetite. Although the intake of protein was more than the requirement, much of the protein was utilised for energy and, as such, wasted.

To summarise, the traditional weaning foods, together with episodes of anorexia caused by illnesses, lead to restricted energy intake in the first year of life. After that, in the second year, the transition from a diet with a relatively high energy concentration, viz. breast milk, to one with low energy concentration leads to intakes of energy which are only just about at maintenance levels for a considerable period of time.

THE ROLE OF INTERCURRENT INFECTIONS

Infections and intercurrent illnesses play an important role in the aetiology of nutritional disorders. The episodes of illness increase after the age of 6 months as the passive immunity derived from the mother begins to decline. The common infectious diseases of childhood, like chickenpox, whooping cough, measles and others usually occur in the first 3 or 4 years of life. Respiratory infections and, in endemic areas, episodes of malaria occur repeatedly after the first 4 months. Diarrhoea is also common and a well-recognised hazard of the weaning period, as indicated by the phrase 'weanling diarrhoea'. Diarrhoeal episodes at the time of weaning are common in several mammals, like the cat and the pig, and in both they are known to be lethal. Several explanations have been put forward to account for weanling diarrhoea. Irritation of the gut by new and unaccustomed foods, change from a liquid to a semi-solid diet and many other factors have been mentioned. But above all, ingestion of contaminants and large numbers of pathogens would appear to be the most important cause according to recent studies in the Gambia. Diarrhoea is now recognised as a major associate of malnutrition.

Each episode of infection causes a slowing of growth and even loss of weight if the illness has been severe. This is followed by a period of catch-up growth during recovery (figure 5.2). If the interval between

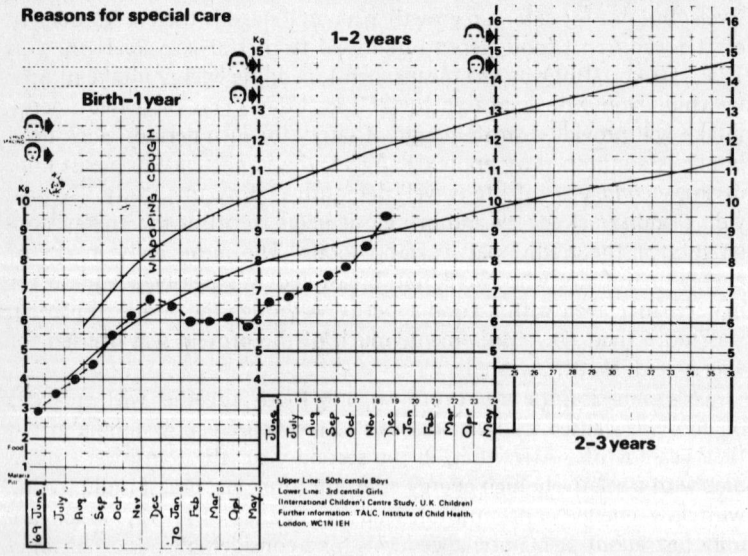

Figure 5.2 Catch-up growth after whooping cough

infections is too short, catch-up growth cannot occur and there is progressive deterioration in the nutritional status. Again the amount of bulk in the diet is an important consideration. If the food contains as little as 1 kcal/g a child weighing 10 kg would need to eat 1 kg of the food daily to consume enough calories. A sick child who is anorexic, coughing or vomiting would need to consume 300-500 g of the food at each meal and this may well be beyond his capacity.

In view of the known effects of illness on the nutritional status of the individual, requirements of protein and energy should not be thought of in terms of physiological requirements alone. The food consumed must provide a substantial cushion for the stress of infection in addition to supplying the physiological requirements of maintenance and growth.

CATCH-UP GROWTH

Growth is a highly sensitive process which requires the optimal functioning of the body's physiological processes together with an adequate supply of nutrients. Any illness, however mild, upsets the delicate balance and growth falters. Under normal circumstances, growth accelerates during recovery and the lost ground is recovered. This period of accelerated growth is known as catch-up growth.

Catch-up growth requires additional nutrients. Observations on infants recovering from protein-calorie malnutrition have shown that such infants gain weight at the rate of 10 g/kg per day compared to normal infants of the same size who grow at the rate of 3.3 g/kg per day. The malnourished infants consumed 169 kcal/kg per day compared to 120 kcal/kg per day in the normals. Thus, assuming that the increased food intake represents the cost of tissue formed, it would appear that about 50-80 kcal are required for the formation of 10 g body weight. Laboratory studies have shown that 3 moles of ATP (adenosine triphosphate) are required for the activation of each amino acid and its attachment by a peptide bond to a protein. Some 6 or more moles of ATP may be used up for each peptide bond which is formed. Each amino acid transported across a cell membrane uses up 3 moles of ATP. Thus, protein synthesis is very expensive in terms of energy requirement, especially when it is realised that for glucose and fat the maximum energy convertible to ATP is between 38 and 40 per cent. The remainder is released as heat. More recent studies indicate that in the case of the child recovering from malnutrition, 1.37 g of protein is being synthesised for every gram of protein deposited. The energy cost of protein synthesis is in the region of 0.9 kcal/g. Further calculations from these baseline data indicate that protein synthesis accounts for about 21 per cent of the energy cost of growth. Thus the energy needs of catch-up growth are heavy and there is a need for concentrated forms of energy and protein in the weanling's diet. The traditional diets, in most instances, are unable to cope with such needs.

LONGITUDINAL STUDIES

The average growth curve derived from cross-sectional studies or from annual measurements of a cohort of children conceals cycles of growth impairment caused by seasonal falls in food supply or illnesses. Studies have therefore been undertaken in which accurate measurements were made of daily food intake of young children over a period of time, maintaining records of illnesses and observing the effects of both on the growth of children. Such studies have been reported from India, Guatemala, Uganda and the Gambia. Together they have thrown further light on the interaction of causative factors in childhood malnutrition. Until recently it was thought that the two clinical syndromes of kwashiorkor and marasmus stemmed from different types of nutritional deficiency. It was believed that kwashiorkor was mainly due to deficiency of protein and that marasmus was caused by inadequate intake of calories. Creation of laboratory models of the two syndromes in animals by the restriction of proteins or total calories gave further support to such hypotheses. Several international meetings under the aegis of UN agencies discussed 'the world protein gap' and explored the possibilities of increasing the production of protein foods. Data from the longitudinal studies mentioned above have helped to rectify some of the concepts regarding infantile malnutrition.

Studies carried out by the National Institute of Nutrition in Hyderabad, India, provided the first evidence on the basis of which the above view was questioned. Three hundred children were observed from birth onwards for varying periods and 90 of them until the age of 3 years. It was found that growth was satisfactory up to the age of 4 months, after which growth curves flattened and there were varying degrees of emaciation. In some it was sufficiently severe to be labelled marasmus. Seven children developed frank kwashiorkor. Analysis of the dietary patterns in these children revealed that there was no difference in types and quantities of food consumed between children who developed kwashiorkor and those who did not. Similarly, there was no qualitative difference in the foods consumed and in the protein : calorie ratio of the diets between cases of kwashiorkor and marasmus or between cases of clinical malnutrition on the one hand and the other growth-retarded children in the community on the other. It was obvious that cases of kwashiorkor and marasmus were the end results of more severe degrees of the same type of protein-calorie deficiency prevalent in the rest of the community. Another revealing observation was that five of seven children who developed kwashiorkor had suffered recurrent bouts of diarrhoea for some days, during which appetite had been lost and food intake reduced. These children were fed their usual foods, but in smaller quantities. In one child chickenpox had preceded kwashiorkor. In one child the onset of kwashiorkor was gradual, with no special precipitating factors. On the basis of their study, the Hyderabad researchers came to the conclusion that during nutritional deficiency growth slows down to adapt to the low intake of nutrients. They further suggested that a breakdown in the physiological process of adaptation produces the clinical picture of kwashiorkor and that the stress of infection is a common cause of such a failure of adaptation. This view gains further support from similar observations made elsewhere.

Metabolic adaptation to inadequate energy intake is mediated by changes in the hormonal pattern. Insulin and cortisol are the two main hormones investigated. Studies in Gambian children showed that fasting plasma cortisol levels were high but insulin levels low in those experiencing faltering growth rates. Furthermore, the insulin : cortisol ratio was strongly correlated with growth velocities. On the other hand, hormonal profiles of pre-school children in Uganda where kwashiorkor is more common showed high levels of plasma insulin.

Investigators at the Infant Malnutrition Unit in Kampala studied 45 children in a rural area from birth to the age of 3 years. The daily intakes of energy and protein were measured and records of illnesses were maintained. Their findings regarding the important role of breast milk in the second year of life, viz. that of calorie density, and the effects of anorexia caused by illness have already been described on page 89. Breastfed children aged 13-18 months consumed 25 per cent more energy than those who were not breast fed. Amongst older children aged 19-24 months, the additional consumption of energy was 17 per cent amongst those who were breast fed. Their work also emphasised the frequency of illness episodes during the weaning period in many developing countries (table 5.2). From this table it is apparent that recurrent illnesses and their influence on appetite may be more important in childhood malnutrition than nutritional deficiency by itself. In a similar study of 110 families in South India, 7325 illness episodes were recorded during a period of 21 months (= 10.6 illnesses per person/year). The majority of illnesses were recorded in children under the age of 5 years.

The role of measles in the aetiology of malnutrition in tropical Africa has been described by Morley in Nigeria. It is not unusual for a child to lose up to 5 per cent of his body weight in a severe attack of measles, especially when there was a weight deficit to begin with. These

Table 5.2 *Total number of illnesses per 100 children*

	Kampala	Newcastle
Upper respiratory tract infections	74	13
Lower respiratory tract infections	258	124
Diarrhoea	107	20
Skin sepsis	160	8
Measles	36	18
Round worms	33	–
Hook worms	48	–
Malaria	257	–

early observations have now been confirmed by other workers. Traditional beliefs about the aetiology of the disease and food taboos related to it make measles one of the commonest precipitating factors of childhood malnutrition in many parts of the Third World.

More recently, studies on the ecology of malnutrition in Gambia have shown that diarrhoeal disease may be as important as measles, if not more. The Gambian workers found that between the ages of 7 and 13 months, children in the study villages suffered from diarrhoea for 6 days in each month. Unlike measles, which is an acute illness, diarrhoea is recurrent and the adverse effects of several episodes of diarrhoea tend to be cumulative. In the Gambia, diarrhoea was found to be almost exclusively the non-dietary element in failure to grow. Bacteriological examination of wells and household water pots showed heavy contamination with faecal coliforms, the average bacterial count being 10^5/ml total organisms and 10^2 *E. coli*/ml of water. Considering that water with coliform counts in excess of 10/100 ml is usually considered unsuitable for drinking, the above counts indicate the extent of contamination. Naturally, this was also reflected in the gruels and other foods used for feeding infants. Freshly cooked food was generally acceptable in quality, but on keeping for half an hour unacceptable levels of pathogens could be detected in the foods. When children with a history of protracted diarrhoea were studied for the bacteriology of the upper bowel, 76 per cent showed bacterial counts of 10^4/ml compared to the upper levels of normal at 10^3. The spectrum of organisms found was also different from the normal bowel flora.

Very similar results were obtained in Guatemala, where a cohort of 45 village children were the subject of a longitudinal study, including the prevalence of diarrhoea. The peak prevalence of diarrhoea was 87 per 100 person-months in the age group 18–23 months. Contamination of water and food was an important element in the transmission of diarrhoeal illness. Bacterial counts in tortillas, the common staple food, were suppressed by cooking, but only temporarily. Within hours they became alarmingly high. Among the illnesses causing loss of weight, diarrhoea, measles and whooping cough produced maximum damage; especially in children who were already underweight. In such children an episode of one of these illnesses could lead to a weight loss of as much as 5 per cent.

The information obtained from the various studies described above has helped to challenge the orthodox view of the aetiology of malnutrition in several ways. It is now widely accepted that in the traditional dietaries the over-riding deficiency is that of calories. Whenever the diets were judged to be low in protein, they were so because the *total* food intake was low. Much of the protein is then burnt to provide energy instead of being utilised as protein. The implication is that had the children consumed a sufficient amount of their usual food to provide the energy requirement, they would have consumed enough protein also.

Secondly, it is now realised that in the past too much emphasis has been put on protein, especially on that of *animal* origin. True, protein is essential, but only like all other essential nutrients. For example, fat-soluble vitamins are essential and deficiency disorders arise when they are not consumed in adequate quantities. But in excess they cause toxic symptoms. Water-soluble vitamins are equally essential. When large quantities are ingested, the body excretes them because, unlike fat-soluble vitamins, a mechanism for excretion exists. In the same way protein is essential, but when consumed in excess the body burns it as calories and excess protein is disposed of. It is of course an uneconomical way of obtaining calories, both financially and biochemically. The yield of ATP from protein is in the range of 32-34 per cent compared to 38-40 per cent with carbohydrates and fats. This change in the status of protein from its exalted position in the past, and the events leading to such re-thinking have been well described by McLaren as 'The great protein fiasco'.

Thirdly, the contribution of infection to malnutrition has hitherto been underestimated. The reasons are obvious. The observed inadequacies of traditional weaning foods, the clinical response to feeding in patients suffering from malnutrition, the creation of laboratory models of kwashiorkor and marasmus, have all helped to generate the view that nutritious food was the only thing that mattered. The above studies from different parts of the world show that the origin of malnutrition rests in two factors: (1) the lack of adequate knowledge and technology at the level of the village home for preparing adequate weaning foods, and (2) lack of knowledge for avoiding the microbial and other pathogens in the environment.

Finally, clinicians and nutritionists have been preoccupied with identifying the biological factors causing malnutrition. Sociocultural factors have not been studied in sufficient detail. For example, the principal care-takers and providers of children are the parents, and the quality of parenting is a crucial determinant of the health and development of children. In a longitudinal study of 334 infants from birth until age 5 years in Mexico, 22 were found to develop a clinically severe form of malnutrition. Environmental factors like family size and structure; sociocultural background of parents; family income; as well as biological characteristics of parents like age, parity, weight and height showed no difference between the affected and control groups. However, there was a marked difference in home stimulation between the two groups. In some instances lack of home stimulation was the first sign of future trouble and its presence was identified at age 6 months, even before malnutrition had occurred. Lack of stimulation acted as an indicator of deficiency in the social environment of the child.

THE ROLE OF INFECTION IN THE AETIOLOGY OF MALNUTRITION

As already noted, the energy cost of protein synthesis is high. An adult synthesising 400 g of protein per day for the normal protein turnover requires 1.4 kcal/g protein or 600 kcal for the purpose. In malnourished children the daily protein turnover is in the range of 15–18 g/kg body weight during the phase of recovery often amounting to 150 g of new tissue being deposited daily. This amount of protein represents a large quantity of energy, which thus becomes an important constraint in protein synthesis.

During infective illnesses, complex changes occur in protein metabolism. There is an increased flux of amino acids from skeletal muscle; phenylalanine, tryptophan, alanine and glutamine move into the extracellular compartment, mainly as a result of increased catabolism in the skeletal muscles, and perhaps also in skin protein. The synthesis of visceral proteins for example in heart and brain is not significantly affected. Also the synthesis of intrahepatic proteins is not altered, but amino acids are utilised at an accelerated rate by the liver for the synthesis of acute phase plasma globulins and for conversion to carbohydrate (gluconeogenesis). Amino acids are also utilised by leucocytes for the synthesis of antibody, gamma-globulin and other factors involved in the immune mechanisms. The caloric needs of the body are also increased under the stress of infection, but because of the accompanying anorexia the consumption of calories is low. The septic patient is unable to mobilise his fat stores or synthesise ketones at a rate fast enough to meet his energy needs. The result is a marked increase in gluconeogenesis from amino acids and an increased breakdown of skeletal muscle to supply these substrates. It is not surprising therefore that the negative nitrogen balance during severe infection can be four times that during starvation. For example, in starvation 4 g of nitrogen are excreted daily in urine, whereas in the septic patient nitrogen excretion may be as much as 15 g/day. As the wasting of body protein continues, the short supply of certain amino acids, such as the branched-chain amino acids, can be rate-limiting. This in turn causes a depletion of host proteins and a reduction in the body's defence mechanisms. Children with clinical malnutrition simply do not have sufficient nutritional reserves to effect the metabolic responses like those described above in well-nourished adults during acute infections.

Similar metabolic responses also occur after elective surgery or injury. In adult patients admitted to hospital for elective surgery weight loss equivalent to between 6 and 8 per cent of bodyweight is not unusual. A general increase in the resting metabolic expenditure of 10-30 per cent above basal has been described after multiple fractures. Increases of 25-45 per cent are known to occur after sepsis and 40-100 per cent after major burns. This increase in the resting metabolic expenditure represents an erosion of body tissues in response to injury or infection and must be recovered from a nourishing diet during convalescence.

Catabolic responses occur in all infectious illnesses regardless of the microbial agent or the presence of symptoms. Even subclinical or silent infections induce stress responses with increased nitrogen excretion in the urine, though naturally the intensity of catabolic response is proportional to the severity of the illness. As a result of such responses the energy requirements of the body are increased and skeletal muscle is catabolised to provide the substrate for energy.

In summary, the metabolic changes during infection are of three types: (1) over-utilisation of nutrients; (2) sequestration of nutrients; and (3) diversion of nutrients. In over-utilisation there is increased utilisation of energy sources like glycogen, mobilisation of amino acids for gluconeogenesis, mobilisation of fat and over-utilisation of vitamins. Sequestration of iron in the liver explains the anaemia of children who have suffered recurrent infections. Nutrient diversion occurs when plasma amino acids are utilised for the synthesis of acute-phase reactant proteins.

The above observations stress the need for change from the orthodox emphasis on food alone to a practical approach in which infective illness receives more importance as the causative and precipitating factor in malnutrition. The diet of the child during illness and in convalescence has not received the attention it deserves. Traditional attitudes like offering light diets for easy digestibility, 'resting the gut', or 'fluids only' persist. The presence of vomiting and anorexia, impaired absorption of nutrients during diarrhoea and even loss of protein in the gut during severe measles add to the difficulty of nursing the febrile child. The reduction of dietary intake during illness can be as serious as the metabolic effects of infection. For example, 23 per cent of rural Guatemalan children showed presence of symptoms on any given day in one study over a period of 7 years. The average reduction of food intake was 175 kcal/day (= 19 per cent intake) and 4.8 g protein per day (= 18 per cent daily intake) in the individual child whilst symptoms lasted.

GUT DYNAMICS IN MALNUTRITION

As we have noted earlier, the gut is working at full capacity during infancy in order to absorb the nutrients required for the rapid growth during that period. Any adverse influences on gut dynamics will affect digestion and absorption of nutrients and will interfere with growth. The epithelial cells of the small intestine are highly differentiated both morphologically and biochemically to carry out the processes of digestion, absorption and transport. These cells, or enterocytes, begin their life cycle in the crypts of the villi and travel to reach the tip as they mature. They are finally sloughed into the gut lumen at the end of their life cycle, which normally lasts from 2 to 5 days.

In the disease kwashiorkor, there is extensive damage to the mucosa of the gut. At the same time there is a reduction in the secretions of the digestive enzymes, notably the secretions of the pancreas. Various forms of malabsorption occur in keeping with these changes. In marasmus, the mucosal structure is generally normal on light microscopy, though various intracellular changes can be seen with the electron microscope. Gut function in children who are marginally undernourished has not been studied extensively. No gross defects in absorption have yet been described in such children. On the other hand, morphological changes in gut mucosa are known to occur in healthy individuals living in a tropical environment. These changes have been described both in the indigenous populations as well as in expatriates living in the tropics. In the latter, the morphological changes are known to revert to normal on return to the home environment. Whether this so-called 'tropical intestine' characterised by stunting of villi and other changes in mucosal architecture, is due to dietary factors or is caused by recurrent non-specific microbial and parasitic insults is not known. Its incidence and its effects on the absorptive capacity of the gut have also not been fully studied.

Alteration of the gut flora in established cases of malnutrition has been described in several countries. The secretions of the upper jejunum in healthy adults and children contain 10^3 bacteria per millilitre except after meals when there is a transient increase due to ingested microorganisms. Studies in the Gambia, Guatemala, Indonesia and in aboriginal Australian children have shown much higher bacterial counts creating 'the contaminated small bowel syndrome'. This contamination of the small bowel reflects the existing contamination of the environment and the ingestion of large numbers of organisms through contaminated food and water. Whether such an alteration of gut flora also occurs in marginally nourished children living in a contaminated environment is not known. Similarly, little is known about the effects of diarrhoeal disease on the absorption and utilisation of nutrients. Preliminary studies in Guatemala indicate that moderate diarrhoea may result in an increased loss of calories in the stool to the extent of 500–600 calories per day.

INTERVENTION PROGRAMMES

Until recently most intervention programmes were based on the free issue of food supplements, chiefly dried skimmed milk powder either by itself or as a 'mix' with other foods. The presence of large surpluses of defatted milk in the West has led to its dumping in the hungry parts of the world under the guise of 'aid'. In many instances the thriving agribusiness in the Western world has lobbied government departments to make sure that conditions attached to the aid programme help to create new markets for their products in the Third World. Food aid has often been used as a lever by donor countries to influence policies and decisions of governments in the Third World. As far as peasant societies are concerned, however, free hand-outs have only given rise to dependency and taken away local initiative.

The whole aspect of intervention at village level is now being reassessed in many countries and several alternative approaches are being developed, aimed at improving knowledge and skills at village level for the production of appropriate weaning foods.

FOOD PRODUCTION: POLICIES AND CONSTRAINTS

It is now generally accepted that the peasant farmer has a vast fund of knowledge and wisdom about efficient low-cost food production acquired over a number of years. By rejecting this experience and seeking to replace it with modern methods planners often throw away the only opportunity they have for developing a locally suited system of agricultural production. Simple additions and improvements in the indigenous farm technology can be more rewarding than the wholesale introduction of new technology. Thus composting and use of farm manure is accepted more easily than chemical fertilisers. Simple methods of conserving the crop and protecting it from rodents and insects can be as fruitful as increasing production with expensive inputs. In the past the emphasis of the planners has been on growing cash crops. A major part of agricultural research effort was devoted to the growing of cash crops, instead of enabling the peasant to become self-sufficient in food. Self-sufficiency through community involvement has to be the main objective of agricultural extension programmes.

Multimixes

Most rural diets tend to be monotonous and are based on the local staple which is the chief source for satisfying hunger. Vegetables, legumes, and occasionally animal foods are used as relishes and to improve the palatability of the diet. The amount of relish consumed depends partly on its availability and partly on custom. As we have seen, this diet is not always adequate to meet the requirements of the weaning period. Recent trends in nutrition science emphasise the use of food mixtures in correct proportions in order to provide a balanced diet. The object is to use multimixes in such a way that up to 7 or 8 per cent of total calories are derived from net utilisable protein. This concept of net dietary protein calories per cent (NdpCal per cent) has been described in Chapter 2 and methods of calculating the amounts of foods to be used as multimixes have been developed. Based on these principles, multimixes from locally available foods have been recommended for different regions of the Third World. If the multimix is consumed in amounts sufficient to provide the daily requirement of calories, then the requirement of protein and other nutrients will be largely taken care of. An important corollary of this concept is the allocation of land for the growing of different crops, such as for example, cereals and pulses, and the rotation of crops. An easy rule of thumb to achieve diversification of crops is to plant a half acre of legumes or pulses for every one and a half acres of grain.

The concept of multimixes is useful not only for the education of the individual parent and farmers but also for promoting community feeding programmes.

THE QUESTION OF BULK IN THE WEANING DIET

The staple foods as well as sources of vegetable protein have a large cellulose and fibre content, which increases their bulk. A child has to consume large quantities of the multimix to obtain his daily requirements, and, as we have seen, during periods of anorexia his capacity for eating may be limited. Hence it is necessary to consider ways and means of increasing the calorie *density* of the weaning food, especially during illness. Fats and oils are the obvious sources of calories, but the traditional foods of many peasant societies do not use much fat in cooking. Exceptions occur in West Africa, where the red palm oil is used in cooking, and in coastal or island communities where the use of coconut or its oil is common. In all other situations, the use of edible oils like cottonseed oil, sunflower oil, or foods with high fat content, like ground nuts, soya beans or sesame seeds, needs to be promoted in the preparation of weaning foods.

PREVENTION OF CONTAMINATION

The problem of microbial contamination of food and water is a difficult one. Its solution is dependent upon the availability of a safe water supply, improvement of standards of cleanliness, personal hygiene and protection of the food from flies. Several studies have noted that bacterial counts in freshly prepared foods are of an acceptable nature, but rise quickly on keeping. At certain times of the year, as in the planting or harvesting seasons, all members of the peasant household must work long hours and the care of the weanling is delegated to an elderly relative or to a sibling. The child is fed on the food cooked by the mother before going to work and kept for several hours. Inevitably it gets contaminated and the incidence of diarrhoea tends to be high during these seasons. Provision of community creches and playgroups where freshly cooked food is offered to the children would be one way of avoiding contamination of food in the village.

In communities where water is available in ample amounts and is safe, the general standard of nutrition and the growth of children tend to be better. This is largely due to a lower incidence of diarrhoeal disease. Thus provision of safe water is an integral part of nutrition intervention. Considering that water is such an essential nutrient, it is surprising how little emphasis has been put on its availability and protection from contamination in all classical nutrition teaching.

Early management of diarrhoea with oral glucose-electrolyte solution in the home will prevent the development of serious dehydration or protracted diarrhoea. Like the concept of NDpCal per cent which has enabled the development of weaning diets from locally available foods, and the concept of energy density, the glucose-electrolyte solution is a major development in medical thinking during the past decade. It has helped to take the management of diarrhoea into the village home. Early recovery will halt the deterioration in the general nutrition of the child which is usually the case when an episode of diarrhoea drags on for several days. Recent experience in several countries has shown that in communities where facilities for prompt oral rehydration exist, the general state of nutrition is better, besides, of course, reduction in mortality from dehydration.

PROVISION OF HEALTH SERVICES

Regular health surveillance of children to identify those at risk will help to identify those families who need advice and help. In many Western countries infant mortality began to decline appreciably only after the large-scale introduction of the infant welfare movement. Many of the important principles of the infant welfare clinic have been adapted to the needs of rural children in the development of the under-5s clinic. Such clinics are a useful way of combining several forms of intervention. Growth supervision, immunisation, nutrition education, treatment of minor ailments, home visiting and identification of those 'at risk' are all combined into one service programme with far-reaching impact on the health of children.

The antenatal and the under-5s clinics are two essential health activities for the regular surveillance of the vulnerable groups in the community. They provide the main foundations for all maternal and child health programmes. They are also activities for which community involvement and participation is usually forthcoming. Thus, they hold the promise of becoming the springboards for other programmes of community development like literacy classes, farmers' clubs, parents' groups, youth activities and so on. Such social groups are often the training grounds for leadership and for larger co-operative efforts by the community. These approaches are further discussed in Chapter 9.

PART-TIME VILLAGE HEALTH WORKERS

Many of the functions of advising parents with regard to multimixes, carrying out regular health surveillance of village children, providing emergency treatment and first aid during acute illness, can be adequately performed by the part-time village health worker. In several projects such a worker has been shown to be successful in raising community awareness about the needs of children and other vulnerable groups. Since such workers are normally selected by the community and are long-time residents of the village, they also act as useful links between health services and the community. The part-time village health worker has an important contribution to make in improving the health and nutrition of village children through intervention at the level of the village home.

FURTHER READING

Cunningham, N. The under-fives' clinic – what difference does it make? *J. Trop. Paed.* (1978), 24, 239-334.

Ebrahim, G. J. Nutrition and its disorders. In *Paediatric Practice in Developing Countries.* Macmillan, Basingstoke and London, 1981, pp. 40-72.

Gopalan, C. Kwashiorkor and marasmus. Evolution and distinguishing features. In McCance, R. A. and Widdowson, E. M. (eds.) *Calorie Deficiency and Protein Deficiency.* J. & A. Churchill, London, 1968.

Gwatkin, D. R., Wilcox, J. R. and Wray, J. D. *Can Health and Nutrition Interventions Make a Difference?* Overseas Development Council, 1717 Massachusetts Avenue, NW, Washington, DC, 1980.

International Union of Nutrition Sciences: Guidelines on policies and procedures for community action and family nutrition programmes. *J. Trop. Ped.* (1980), 26, 156-66.

Mata, L. J. *The Children of Santa Maria Cauque: a prospective field study of health and growth.* MIT Press, Cambridge Mass, and London, UK, 1978.

McLaren, D. S. The great protein fiasco. *Lancet* (1974), 2, 93-6.

Morley, D. C. The Under-fives' clinic – comprehensive child care. In *Paediatric Priorities in the Developing World.* Butterworths, London, 1973, pp. 316-40.

Rowland, M. G. M. and Whitehead, R. G. The epidemiology of protein-energy-malnutrition in children in a West African village community. Medical Research Council, Dunn Nutrition Unit, Cambridge (u.d. mimeo).

Schuften, C. Nutrition intervention programmes for rural areas: African experiences. *J. Trop. Ped.* (1981), 27, 177-81.

Waterlow, J. C. (Ed.) *Nutrition of Man.* Churchill Livingstone, London, 1981.

Chapter 6

Protein-Energy Malnutrition

Protein-energy malnutrition (PEM) is currently the most widespread and serious health problem of children in the world. At any time approximately 100 million children suffer from the moderate or severe forms of PEM. In any one country the prevalence rates will be influenced by the season, the availability of food, the incidence of infection, and the state of development of the health services. As can be expected, the peak incidence is immediately after epidemics of infectious illnesses and diarrhoea or in the 'hungry' months. Results of community surveys in the past 10 years in 17 different countries and involving 173 000 children reveal an aggregate prevalence rate of 20 per cent (Table 6.1).

Table 6.1 *The prevalence of childhood malnutrition*

Area	No. of surveys	No. of children examined (thousands)	Severe forms		Moderate forms	
			Range (%)	Median (%)	Range (%)	Median (%)
Latin America	11	109	0.5– 6.3	1.6	3.5–32.0	18.9
Africa	7	25	1.7– 9.8	4.4	5.4–44.9	26.5
Asia	7	39	1.1–20.0	3.2	16.0–46.4	31.2
Total	25	173	0.5–20.0	2.6	3.5–46.4	18.9

Taking the median values, an approximate estimation of the geographical distribution of childhood malnutrition can be made in Table 6.2. The figures in Table 6.2 provide only an estimate of the size of the problem. Exact statistics will not become available until health services of the developing countries are able to achieve universal coverage of the population and efficient methods for the collection of health data are established. At present only 20 per cent of rural populations receive

Table 6.2 *Geographical distribution of childhood malnutrition*

Area	Population aged 0-5 years (millions)	No. of children with PEM (millions)	
		Severe	Moderate
South America	46	0.7	8.8
Africa	61	2.7	16.3
Asia	206	6.6	64.4
Total	313	10.0	89.5

health care on a regular basis, and health coverage of the urban poor is even less in some countries. Hence most health statistics are rudimentary. Thus community surveys at regular intervals provide the only means of measuring the size of the problem. As a result of such surveys it is possible to generalise that at any time 10 per cent of the children in an average peasant community will show signs of growth failure and some of them will have clinical signs of malnutrition. Only 24 per cent of children in such communities show adequate growth, and the remaining 66 per cent experience faltering of growth from time to time.

The level of preschool (1-5 years) mortality in a country may also indicate the prevalence of childhood malnutrition. This is because of the well-known synergism between undernutrition and infection. The preschool mortality in the average developing country is about 40 times that of western countries, which again reveals the size of the problem of malnutrition. Recently, in a study of the patterns of childhood mortality in 13 areas in South America, sponsored by the Pan American Health Organisation, 7318 deaths in children between the ages of 1 and 4 years were studied. Malnutrition was found to be the primary cause of death in 9 per cent (range 0-18 per cent) and an associated cause of death in 48.4 per cent (range 0-61 per cent). The general conclusion was that malnutrition was directly or indirectly responsible for 57.4 per cent of deaths of children aged 1-4 years.

CLASSIFICATION AND DEFINITION

It is paradoxical that such a widespread, serious and extensively studied form of nutritional disorder still continues to be a controversial subject in almost every aspect. This is especially so with regard to classification and pathogenesis. The reason is that the presenting features of nutritional deficiency vary from one part of the world to another, due mainly to the great variation in the nutrient content of the diet, the prevalence of antecedent illnesses, the variability of the host, and the time over which the causative factors operate. Two distinct clinical syndromes have been described, viz. kwashiorkor and marasmus, and represent the severe forms of PEM. They occupy the two ends of a spectrum with a mixture of the clinical features of both in between. The biochemical features also form a spectrum though they are more evident in kwashiorkor than in marasmus. It is not unusual to find that a child diagnosed as suffering from kwashiorkor shows the typical features of marasmus after the oedema (see 'Clinical features') subsides, while a child with nutritional marasmus often develops oedema and progresses to marasmic kwashiorkor.

Of the two classical syndromes, kwashiorkor has received a great deal of interest and attention because of the striking clinical features and extensive changes in the body's chemistry. However, there are now clear indications that marasmus is on the increase, especially in the city slums and shanty towns of the developing countries. The rapid decline in breast feeding has a great deal to do with this. Moreover, since marasmus usually occurs at a younger age than kwashiorkor, its long-term effects are more severe. In both forms of malnutrition, recognition at an early stage is important in order to avoid the serious after-effects of established malnutrition. Hence there has been great interest in accurate classification and especially in identifying early signs.

Mild-to-moderate malnutrition

In defining the stages of malnutrition, two processes have to be taken into account. These are: (1) the period over which malnutrition occurs, so as to decide whether it is acute or chronic, or acute on chronic. Acute forms chiefly affect body weight more than height, whereas in the chronic form both height and weight are affected. (2) The aetiological factors. The classical explanation that kwashiorkor is due to protein deficiency with relatively adequate energy supply while marasmus is due to the overall deficiency of proteins and calories arose out of the observations that in countries where roots, tubers and plantain (all with 1–2 per cent protein) form the staple foods kwashiorkor is more common. This view has been challenged, as we saw in the previous section, and the role of infection has come to be emphasised in the aetiology of malnutrition.

In every locality the identification of the important aetiological factors is necessary for instituting early intervention. When food is inadequate, the organism adapts first of all by reducing growth and the clinical signs are those of such adaptation. Thus, weight gain slows down, and so weight for age has been commonly used to assess the degree of mild to moderate malnutrition. Those children who weigh less than the mean weights of children in their age group are thus called 'wasted' and the degree of wasting is an indication of the degree of malnutrition they have suffered. A common difficulty is that in most cases parents do not know the ages of their children. Height for age also suffers from the same difficulty. Thus there is a need for age-independent criteria of malnutrition. It has been suggested that the ratio weight/height may overcome this difficulty besides providing a sensitive measure of wasting. Refinements have been added to this measure in the form of regression lines and various indices like weight/height^2 or weight/height$^{1.6}$. One may question the value of these complexities which require mathematical manipulation.

Reduced growth as a consequence of adaptation to lack of food also affects height. Weight can swing up and down, but obviously this is not the case with height. All that happens is that growth in height slows down and the individual will end up short. Those children whose heights are less than the mean heights of children in their age group are called 'stunted'. Catch-up growth in both height and weight can occur if the slowing of growth was temporary, as for example after an acute illness. If dietary deficiency is prolonged, full catch-up does not occur and the deficit in height becomes fixed and permanent. Thus deficits of height indicate long-standing malnutrition.

Besides growth in height and weight, the body compartments most affected in malnutrition are those of energy reserve – subcutaneous fat and the protein store of skeletal muscle. Measuring these two body compartments can shed extra light on the pathophysiological mechanisms. Thus, in malnutrition muscle is wasted not only because of lack of protein in the diet, but because muscle is used up to supply energy. Deficient muscle with adequate body fat will be one indication of protein deficiency. Conversely, adequate muscle with lack of fat suggests lack of energy reserve.

The adaptive changes to dietary deficiency are not always successful. For example, we know that undernourished individuals have a predisposition to infectious illnesses. Diarrhoeal disease is not only more prevalent in undernourished children, but also tends to be more severe. In one study of village children aged between 6 and 32 months in Nigeria it was found that the frequency of diarrhoea during the rainy season was greatest amongst children who were described as 'wasted' (i.e. < 80 per cent of weight/height). Such children suffered 47 per cent more episodes of diarrhoea. Pre-existing malnutrition affected the duration of diarrhoea which was 79 per cent longer in 'wasted' children compared to well-nourished controls. In children who were under-weight (< 75 per cent weight/age) the duration of diarrhoea was 33 per cent longer and in stunted (< 90 per cent height/age) children it was 37 per cent longer compared to those who were well-nourished. In Zaire, childhood infections, especially measles, had occurred in more than half the children in the weeks immediately preceding an outbreak of kwashiorkor. Associated deficiencies besides those of protein and calories also occur with malnutrition. Hence in identifying early malnutrition it is useful to remember that the differing proportions of protein and calories in the diet, the duration of malnutrition, the associated deficiency of other nutrients, and the effects of infectious illnesses together give rise to a wide spectrum of signs and symptoms. The presence of intestinal parasites may also contribute to the typical pattern of malnutrition encountered in a given locality. For example, heavy hookworm infection may contribute to loss of iron as well as protein in the gut; *Strongyloides* infection also acts in a similar manner with added malabsorption, and giardiasis causes impaired absorption.

A new twist has been added to a complex situation by the trend of urban migration and rapid urban growth in most developing countries. The new social problems of unemployment, the need to change from subsistence to cash economy and a deteriorating family life, added to the promotion of a variety of 'junk' foods and beverages, means that multiple deficiencies occur on a background of protein and energy lack.

The Need for Simplification

Such a complex situation has led to a variety of methods of classification. Such methods, however useful as research tools, cannot be easily taught to auxiliaries and village health workers, for whom a more simplified and action-oriented approach is necessary. With this need in mind, several simple methods of measuring nutritional status have been evolved. The Wellcome classification is one such simple method for the diagnosis of clinical malnutrition.

Wellcome classification

Weight (% of standard)	Oedema Present	Absent
80–60	Kwashiorkor	Undernourished
< 60	Marasmic kwashiorkor	Marasmus

For children within the community who are at risk of mild–moderate malnutrition a similar simple tool for the selection of early cases is required. The Gomez classification was first suggested in the late 1950s as a method of diagnosing mild-moderate forms of malnutrition in the community and for the early identification of marasmus. The classification is based on weights of healthy American children under the age of 5 years, and the fiftieth percentile is taken as the standard. Malnutrition is graded into three degrees of increasing severity according to the percentage reduction in weight from the standard.

Gomez classification

First-degree malnutrition	< 80% of the standard
Second-degree malnutrition	< 70% of the standard
Third-degree malnutrition	< 60% of the standard

The Gomez classification has been criticised on two counts. Firstly, it does not take height into consideration. Secondly, in some communities more than half the children fall in the category of third-degree malnutrition, and health workers doubted whether the growth standards of one community were applicable to another. With further experience it is now realised that the place on the growth chart where a child's weight falls is not so important as the shape of his growth curve compared to the standard. This knowledge has helped to remove a great deal of controversy and contributed to the spread of weight charts in most countries of the Third World. When Morley described the first weight chart in Nigeria it carried two curves. The upper curve represented mean weights of children from the upper social class and the lower curve did the same for the lower social class. Since then there has been considerable debate with regard to local standards, definition of 'normal' children and so on. This controversy delayed the development of local weight charts. When it was realised that it was the *shape* of the child's weight curve as compared to normal which was important, and not the actual weight, the use of weight charts based on the Harvard standards received a great boost. More recently a working party convened by the World Health Organization has developed a weight chart for international use (figure 6.1) based on American data. In these charts the upper lines represent the 97th and 50th percentiles respectively. The lower lines are 3rd percentile, −3 standard deviation and −4 standard deviation respectively. Thus, further development in the concept first proposed by Gomez and colleagues has facilitated the regular use of weight charts in children's clinics in many countries.

Present experience shows that it is possible to train auxiliaries and even lesser-trained health personnel in the charting and interpretation of growth records. In the present state of development of health services even these are not available in all areas and the new trend is to

110 Nutrition in Mother and Child Health

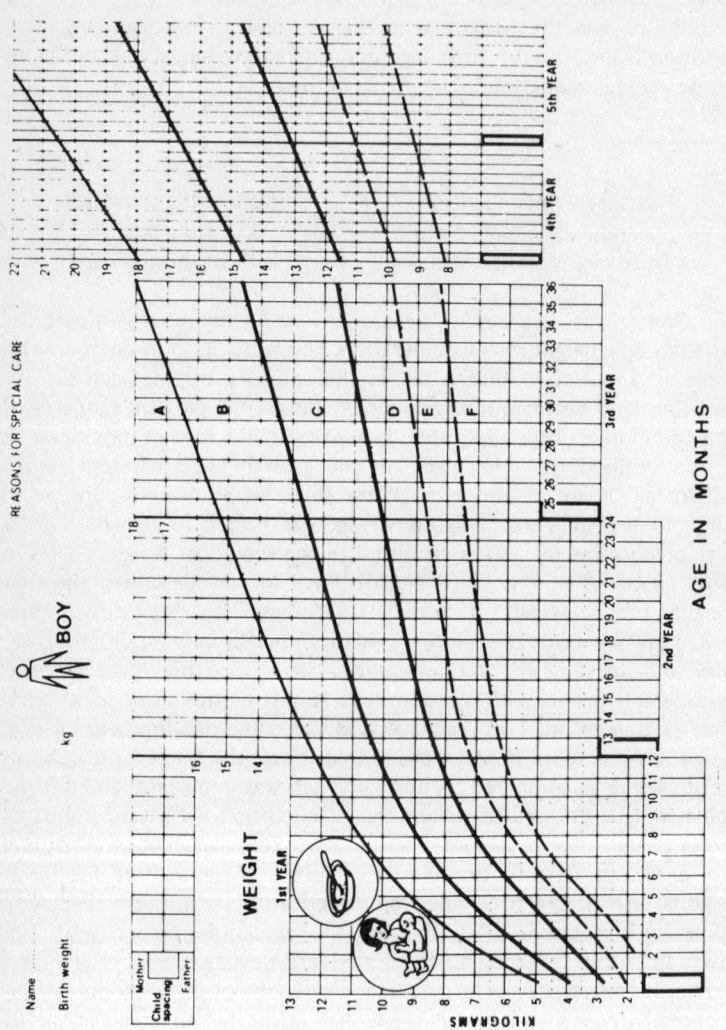

Figure 6.1 Weight chart for international use

train part-time village health workers who are not always literate. A yet simpler way of assessing nutritional status of children is therefore required. Circumference of the mid-arm as an indicator of muscle mass has been used as one of the parameters for measuring nutritional status. It is known that in the normal child between the ages of 1 and 5 years the arm circumference changes very little. Here then is a parameter which is age-independent. The first practical use of this concept was made during the Biafran war for selecting malnourished individuals in the refugee camps for intensive rehabilitation. The arm circumference was compared with the height of the individual and grades of malnutrition were identified in accordance with the percentage reduction in the arm circumference. More recently, Shakir has shown in Baghdad children that measurement of the arm circumference was a useful tool for diagnosing malnutrition. Children whose arm circumference was less than 75 per cent of the standard also had a body weight less than 60 per cent of the Harvard standard in nine cases out of ten in his series. The practical value of this observation is that primary-school children and illiterate village health workers can be trained to use a string or a strip of plastic with a mark and colours in green (over 14.0 cm), yellow (12.5–14.0 cm) and red (less than 12.5 cm) for assessing malnutrition in village children (figures 6.2 and 6.3).

Experience in several countries has shown the practical usefulness

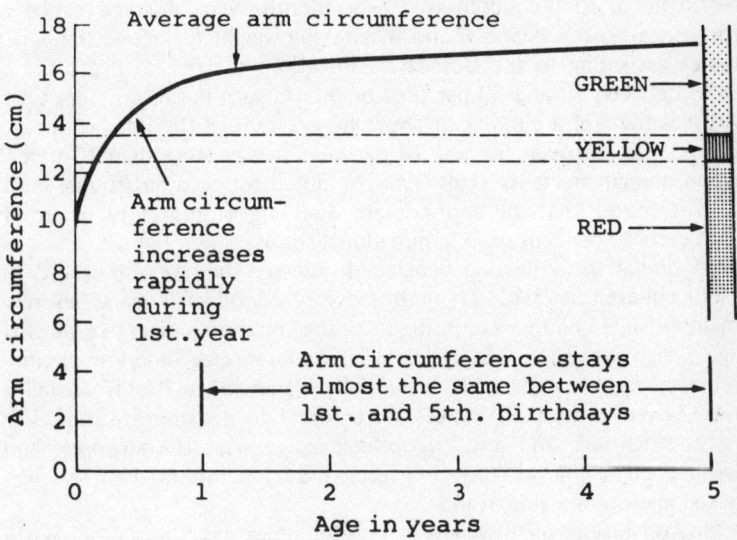

Figure 6.2   The mid-arm circumference as a measure of nutritional status

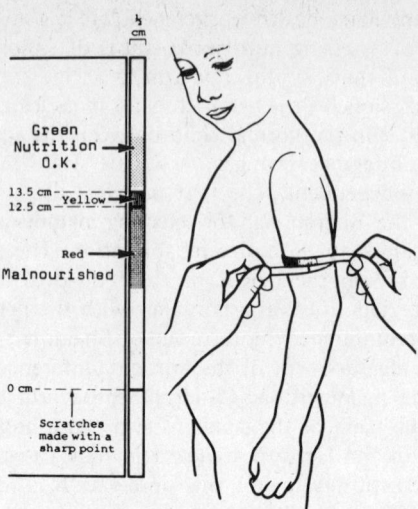

Figure 6.3 Measuring the mid-arm circumference

of the above methods of measuring less severe forms of malnutrition. In the Narangwal study conducted in fourteen villages in the Punjab, North India, 3000 children aged 1-36 months were observed regularly for several years. It was found that taking weight for age as the parameter according to the Gomez classification, the risk of death for a child between 70 and 80 per cent of the Harvard mean was more than 4 times that for a child at or above 80 per cent of the Harvard mean. For a child between 60 and 70 per cent it was more than 10 times. When annual mortality rates were computed for each nutritional level it was found that an approximate doubling of mortality occurred with each 10 per cent drop in nutritional status.

A similar study in rural Bangladesh assessed the risk of mortality in 2019 children aged 13-23 months over a period of 2 years. Severely malnourished children according to all the common indices like weight/age, weight/height, height/age, arm circumference/age and arm circumference/height experienced substantially higher (3- to 7-fold) mortality rates. Even though all indices were found to discriminate mortality risks weight/age and arm circumference/age were the strongest and weight/height the weakest. For each index, a threshold of risk was noted instead of a gradation.

In conclusion, birth weight is a useful indicator of mortality risks in the neonatal period and the first half of infancy. In the first 3 years of life, weight/age can effectively identify those children who are at risk of death. After the age of 1 year and up to the age of 5, the arm circumference is a useful quick technique for identifying those at risk. Children who are both wasted and stunted face greatly increased danger and should be carefully supervised.

CLINICAL FEATURES

In the early stage of malnutrition clinical signs are few and even absent, and diagnosis requires both biochemical tests and anthropometric measurements.

In the severe forms, growth failure is obvious. In addition, activity is reduced so that the child is listless and apathetic or irritable. Because of this irritability communication between the child and the parents is minimal, and often resentment builds up. There is also discoloration of hair and skin, anaemia of varying severity, signs of associated deficiencies and presence of infection.

Kwashiorkor

Kwashiorkor (figure 6.4) presents with failure to thrive, oedema, apathy, anorexia, diarrhoea and discoloration of the skin and hair.

The general appearance may be that of typical 'sugar baby', with chubby features and bloated body, so that at the time parents may think the child is doing well, and they cannot be convinced that he is malnourished.

Failure in growth is marked and weight is reduced in spite of the presence of oedema. Varying degrees of muscle wasting are present. The discoloration of hair and skin gives the child a characteristic 'red baby' appearance. In addition, various forms of skin disorder can also occur. These can vary from the characteristic 'flaky paint' dermatoses to fissures and at times raw ulcerating areas chiefly at the flexures and the buttocks.

Oedema is the characteristic clinical sign of kwashiorkor. It appears first on the dorsum of the feet and ankles and spreads upwards to involve the rest of the body. Oedema fluid can represent 5–20 per cent of body weight so that change in the appearance of the child when the fluid is lost can be striking.

Another major characteristic is the change in personality. Most children with kwashiorkor are apathetic or extremely irritable and miserable. Marked improvement occurs on treatment, and many clinicians stress that the return of the smile is the first sign of improvement.

Physiological functions of the various systems are markedly disturbed,

Nutrition in Mother and Child Health

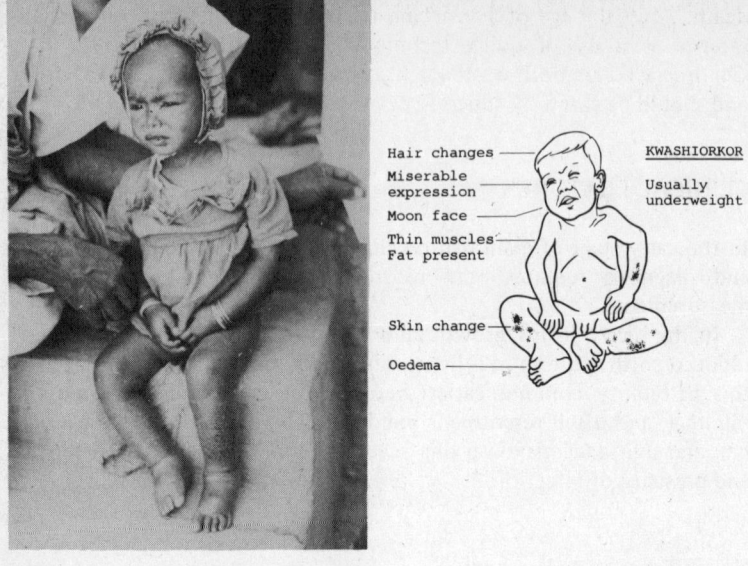

Figure 6.4 Characteristic features of kwashiorkor

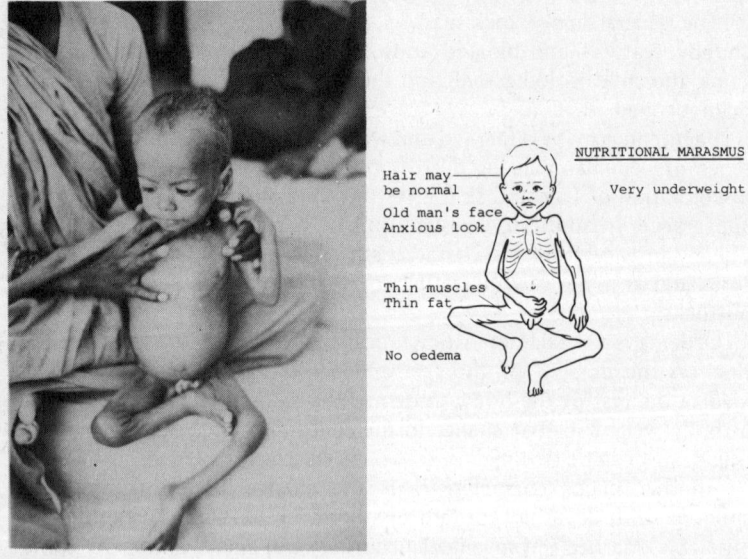

Figure 6.5 Characteristic features of marasmus

with diarrhoea, electrolyte disturbance, circulatory insufficiency, metabolic imbalance and poor renal function. Hence the child with kwashiorkor should be thought of as an emergency in need of intensive medical and nursing care, and not just simply malnourished.

Marasmus (figure 6.5)

This usually occurs in younger children, with failure to thrive. Affected children are short and light for their age. In appearance they are shrunken and wizened due to lack of subcutaneous fat. Until recently kwashiorkor had aroused maximum interest and attention, but it is now increasingly realised that marasmus is a fast-growing disease of the large urban slums and shanty towns in the cities of the Third World. The sharp increase in bottle feeding amongst the urban poor and the new migrants to the cities is largely responsible for the increase in the incidence of marasmus. Since the slums and shanty towns are also the 'septic fringes' of the cities, the marasmic child commonly suffers from infections of all sorts, though more commonly respiratory and diarrhoeal illnesses.

ASSOCIATED DEFICIENCIES

Nutritional deficiency is very rarely restricted to just one or two nutrients. As a rule the deficiency is generalised so that, besides clinical signs of protein and calorie deficiency, there also exist signs of vitamin and other deficiencies.

Many of the illnesses which precipitate protein-calorie malnutrition also provoke loss of nutrients from the body in the same way as they cause a negative nitrogen balance. The type of local food staple, the age of the child, and the time over which the child's diet has been insufficient also help to determine the severity and the nature of associated deficiencies, the most common of which are those of the fat-soluble and water-soluble vitamins and of iron.

Xerophthalmia

In the rice-eating countries of South East Asia, deficiency of vitamin A is endemic and is commonly associated with protein-energy malnutrition. In Indonesia about three-quarters of all cases of kwashiorkor are reported to also have xerophthalmia. In Thailand the incidence is 40 per cent, but in East and West Africa and in the West Indies the reported incidence is only about 1 per cent. Clinical deficiency is only the tip of the iceberg, because in endemic areas children with PEM but no clinical eye signs invariably have low levels of vitamin A and depleted liver stores of the vitamin. Presence of eye lesions therefore indicates a long-standing deficiency and is often a danger signal, since the mortality from PEM in such cases is about four times that of children who have no ocular lesions.

Rickets

Rickets is a common finding in cases of PEM from the urban slums and inner-city areas. It is more common in the younger child suffering from marasmus than in the older child suffering from kwashiorkor. Rickets, like xerophthalmia, has been more commonly reported from South East Asia, where prevalence rates of 15–18 per cent have been recorded. It is a rare finding in East and West Africa and in the West Indies. In endemic areas malnourished children without clinical rickets have low blood levels of the active form of vitamin D.

Vitamin B deficiency

Laboratory tests show that children with PEM have depleted stores of the water-soluble vitamins, chiefly those of the B group. In many cases there are visible manifestations of deficiency disease. The effects of protein deficiency on the mucosal lining of the mouth, skin and gastrointestinal tract may alter the classic manifestations of B-complex deficiency. Many vitamins act as co-enzymes in several key metabolic reactions in the cell. Their deficiency, together with the deficiency of protein and calories, can seriously disrupt cell function. Supplementation with vitamins during treatment is essential in order to replenish tissue stores and to ensure optimal function of the new tissue generated during growth.

Anaemia

Anaemia is also a common accompaniment of protein-calorie malnutrition. The commonest form of anaemia is of the iron deficiency type, which is as expected, since iron deficiency is so widespread in the tropics. But there is very little response to iron therapy until such time as recovery from malnutrition also begins. In several countries the anaemia is reported to respond better to folic acid and B_{12} than to iron.

Hence during treatment it is important to administer several haematinics, the more so because treatment is usually based on an artificial formula containing high energy and protein, and not on a complete food as such.

PATHOLOGICAL FEATURES AND CHANGES IN METABOLISM

As the fat stores of the body are consumed and muscle tissue depleted total body water increases as a percentage of body weight. A direct relationship can be demonstrated between weight deficit and total body water. A proportionate increase occurs in the extracellular fluid. On recovery, some of the excess extracellular fluid is taken up by the regenerating cells and some is lost by diuresis.

As the tissue cells break down, potassium and nitrogen are lost in equal proportions initially. Later on there is increased loss of potassium in diarrhoeal stools causing a cellular deficit of potassium. The total body protein is severely reduced, ranging from 55 to 80 per cent (average 59 per cent) of normal. Non-collagen protein is depleted more than collagen protein. Muscle mass is greatly diminished and may be only 30 per cent of normal for age. Similarly, in marasmus, body fat may fall as low as 5 per cent of total body weight, compared to the normal of 19 per cent.

Changes in the digestive system

LIVER

A fatty liver is characteristic of kwashiorkor. The fat content of the liver may be as high as 50 per cent of the total wet weight. As recovery occurs, fat gradually disappears. Electron microscopy of liver tissue obtained by biopsy reveals that after 3 weeks of treatment on a balanced diet the liver cells are still not visibly normal, even though serum protein levels have reached normal levels. Recognisable liver pathology can be identified even after 10–12 weeks of treatment. Total recovery eventually occurs and liver biopsy 5 years later on light microscopy has shown no signs of residual damage. There are two obvious reasons for the fatty liver. There is an increased flux of fatty acids from adipose tissue for the production of energy. At the same time there is decreased hepatic synthesis of β-lipoproteins which normally transport triglycerides from the liver. The synthesis of the apoprotein part of this fat-transporting mechanism is particularly sensitive to lack of protein in the diet.

PANCREAS

There is a marked atrophy of the acinar cells, and exocrine secretion is reduced in keeping with the atrophic changes. Enzyme activity of the pancreatic juice has been reported to be as low as 50 per cent of normal. Recovery takes place within the first few days of instituting treatment. Investigation of B cell function reveals that in both kwashiorkor and marasmus insulin secretion is abnormally low after oral administration of glucose. Improvement occurs after 3-6 weeks of treatment, though there are instances where an abnormal response persisted up to 10 months after recovery from malnutrition.

GASTROINTESTINAL TRACT

Striking morphological changes occur in the jejunum, especially in kwashiorkor. In particular, villous atrophy may be severe. Enzyme activity is reduced within the cells in keeping with the morphological changes. The enzymes most affected are the ones located in the brush border. Of these, lactase has been studied extensively because it is more severely affected and because most diets used for recovery are based on milk and contain large quantities of lactose. Besides these morphological changes, the small intestine also suffers from bacterial overgrowth with invasion of the proximal gut by the bacterial flora of the distal part of the small intestine. Malabsorption of fat has been correlated with bacterial degradation of bile salts so that the concentration of conjugated bile salts in the gut lumen falls below the critical level necessary for forming micelles with fat.

Some atrophy of the gastric mucosa is common in the majority of cases. Fasting gastric pH is often in the neutral range. Thus the function of the stomach acid as a barrier to intestinal contamination is much reduced. This is supported by the observation that fasting stomach contents in children suffering from PEM have high bacterial and fungal counts.

The changes in gut morphology, together with reduction in the amounts of pancreatic enzymes and bacterial overgrowth of the small gut as well as parasitic disease, are together responsible for the common occurrence of diarrhoea in malnutrition. Impairment of absorption is also likely, but, in most cases, is not severe enough to interfere with recovery. For example, up to 33 g of fat containing unsaturated fatty acids is tolerated daily by malnourished children. Clinical experience with diets containing large quantities of vegetable fat supports this observation and cottonseed oil is now a common ingredient of many dietary regimens. With regard to protein digestion, it has been found that even though faecal nitrogen excretion in malnourished children is on average twice the normal, there is no serious malabsorption of nitrogen. More than three-quarters of the nitrogen in the diet is absorbed and is usually sufficient to allow the initiation of a cure except in very severe diarrhoea. Intolerance of lactose can present a serious problem at times, but even here the incidence of practical difficulties with feeding is small (less than 10 per cent). Thus, knowledge of the alteration in digestion and absorption is helpful in dealing with complications when they arise, but these are rare and in most cases it is possible to treat and rehabilitate children suffering from malnutrition without the need for sophisticated laboratory support.

HEART

The heart muscle suffers in the general atrophy of all muscle tissue. Cardiac output is reduced in accord with the reduced body metabolism. Institution of treatment, by stimulating metabolism, can often precipitate congestive cardiac failure. The salt content of the therapeutic diet and presence of anaemia may contribute to congestive cardiac failure.

HAEMOPOIETIC SYSTEM

A mild to moderate anaemia is a common accompaniment of PEM. Deficiency of nutrients such as protein, iron and folic acid, in addition to bone marrow depression due to infection, are all undoubtedly involved in the aetiology of the anaemia. Parasitic infections such as malaria and hookworm are also of relative importance in the tropics where childhood malnutrition is common. The fall in haemoglobin is related to reduction in the erythrocyte mass which commences with tissue wasting and loss of body weight. Megaloblastic changes in the bone marrow frequently occur and in some areas, e.g. the Sudan, the anaemia is reported to respond to folic acid administration. In the first few days of treatment, with regeneration of plasma proteins and the expansion of plasma volume, the concentration of haemoglobin may fall further, thereby accentuating the anaemia.

MUSCLE

The muscle compartment of the body comprises a large mass of protein which is both labile and sensitive to dietary changes. Muscle wasting is an early result of PEM. At recovery the average muscle mass is usually about twice that during the malnourished state. Muscle and fat biopsies in malnourished Peruvian infants at the time of admission and again 4–9 months later, after recovery, show that there is a gross reduction of muscle cell size in malnourished infants. Improvement takes place with recovery, but the cell size continues to remain subnormal after recovery. Thus clinical recovery does not always reflect cellular maturity.

BRAIN AND THE NERVOUS SYSTEM

Research in the effects of malnutrition on the brain encounters several difficulties. There is the virtual inaccessibility of the brain for study. Secondly, our ignorance of the physical basis of higher mental function is such that it is impossible to relate structural change to function. Thirdly, the important effect of environmental stimulation on intellectual ability makes it difficult to untangle the effects of lack of stimulation from that of undernutrition, since often the two co-exist. However, animal experiments together with observations on long-term effects of malnutrition in children have helped to identify several basic principles. The vulnerability of the growing brain to periods of malnutrition is now widely accepted. The period of growth of the human brain corresponding to a 'vulnerable period' in animal experiments would seem to extend from about mid-pregnancy to the second birthday.

The type of damage suffered is closely related to the timetable of development, and will depend upon the developmental events at the time of the insult. Growth impairment is more in the form of failure of assembly of certain components (or their sizes or numbers) rather than destructive lesions. Thus, the mature product may turn out to be not only deficient or small, but also distorted. Metabolic and biochemical functions of the brain may be altered, and several of these, like catecholamine metabolism, are related to higher mental function. Hence at a time when a large number of components are being formed and assembled, the vulnerability is greatly increased, as for example during the period of the growth spurt of the brain.

The timetable of brain development is such that many of the events have possibly only a single opportunity to occur. If conditions are not optimal at a given time, that opportunity is lost and compensation may be difficult. This means that different parts of the brain may be affected to a variable extent by the same insult. The cerebellum, for example, is selectively affected and within the cerebellum certain structures bear the major brunt.

How do the above principles derived from laboratory studies and animal experiments relate to the situation in the human? In one study, 74 Jamaican school-age boys, who had suffered severe malnutrition in the first 2 years of life, were compared with male siblings closest in age and classmates or neighbours matched for age and sex. The IQ was found to be significantly lower in all aspects of measurements in the index cases, and in particular the full scale and verbal IQ. In this study, however, no relationship could be established between the level of IQ and the age at which malnutrition occurred. Another study from South Africa followed up 20 children who were grossly undernourished in infancy, until they were 15-18 years old. All the children scored low on full scale and verbal quotient. Other tests showed a marked disturbance of visual-motor perception in 17 of these children. Even though a catch-up in height had occurred in all the children, the difference in head circumference as compared to controls got worse. The persistence of low IQ well into the teens indicates the permanence of damage to mental function. Similar studies from Uganda have confirmed these observations and have related the mental deficit to the chronic undernutrition suffered by such children.

To conclude, if malnutrition is a measure of disadvantage and of deficiencies in the child's environment, then the damage or distorted growth suffered by the delicate nervous system represents a tragic outcome of such disadvantage. The stunting of brain growth condemns the victims of malnutrition to a lifetime of failure of learning.

Metabolic changes

CARBOHYDRATE METABOLISM

Low blood sugar is a common accompaniment of PEM. Two types of hypoglycaemia have been identified – asymptomatic, from which recovery occurs with feeding; and the profound irreversible type, associated with severe malnutrition, hypothermia or infection. As a general rule, if the child has hypothermia it is almost certain that hypoglycaemia is also present.

FAT METABOLISM

Fat malabsorption is common in PEM, but the degree is rarely serious enough to cause steatorrhoea. Probably the most serious result of fat malabsorption is the impairment of absorption of fat-soluble vitamins. It has been found that vegetable fats are better absorbed than animal fats and this is the rationale behind the use of cottonseed oil as a source of energy in the treatment of kwashiorkor.

PROTEIN METABOLISM

Protein digestion, though inefficient because of low levels of pancreatic trypsin, is sufficient for recovery to occur when an adequate diet is being fed. On average, absorption of nitrogen from a milk-based diet is 70-80 per cent as compared to 90 per cent in the normal child. Similarly, in the absence of complicating infection, nitrogen is well retained, being in the range of 20-40 per cent of the intake. Thus, protein repletion through a greatly enhanced anabolism is usual as soon as sufficient protein is given. Nitrogen retention continues to be high until a normal growth rate has been attained.

Albumin synthesis and its level in plasma are very sensitive to protein intake. There is an immediate fall when dietary deficiency occurs, and a rise when the deficiency is corrected. Serum albumin levels are also sensitive to infection. The longitudinal study of Ugandan children referred to earlier showed that a combination of respiratory infection, diarrhoea and malaria caused a dramatic fall in serum albumin.

Defence mechanisms

The child with malnutrition is susceptible to infection. The body's defences are unable to mount an adequate response to microbial challenge so that the mildest infection tends to spread and become generalised. In severe cases the clinical response to infection, like fever and phagocytosis, may be absent and the first sign of widespread infection may be sudden deterioration in the general condition, refusal to take food and hypothermia.

Studies of the body's defence mechanisms reveal adequate capacity for humoral immunity. Thus immunoglobulin levels in the blood are normal and there are normal numbers and proportions of B lymphocytes, which produce immunoglobulins. Secretory IgA in salivary and nasopharyngeal secretions, and in the gastrointestinal tract, is reduced and does not rise in response to antigenic challenge. This impairment of secretory antibody response in malnourished children explains their slow recovery from enteric infections and viral illnesses like measles. In contrast to humoral immunity, cellular immunity (T-cell function) is profoundly impaired. T-lymphocytes are reduced in number to about a third of normal and various tests of their functions also show impairment. In keeping with the lowered cellular immunity, all lymphoid organs show atrophy, especially the thymus. A useful clinical sign for assessing the involution of lymphoid organs is the size of the tonsils in malnourished children. Phagocytic function is also inefficient and several workers have emphasised its correlation with iron deficiency, especially lower levels of serum transferrin.

MANAGEMENT

The objectives of treatment are:

(1) to achieve rapid regeneration of tissues and institute cure of the malnutrition;
(2) to treat complications and reduce case fatality – the present mortality rates are as high as 20–40 per cent;
(3) to achieve rehabilitation on a well-balanced solid diet;
(4) to prevent relapse and future deterioration, through education of the parents;
(5) to achieve long-term follow-up with a view to helping the child and his family.

The principle of treatment is to raise the nutritional level of the child by administering adequate calories, proteins, minerals and vitamins and to get him to eat a well-balanced diet prepared from local foods in as short a time as possible.

During recovery a linear relationship can be demonstrated between velocity of weight gain and the intake of energy, varying from virtually no weight gain at 100 kcal/kg per day to a maximum at 200 kcal/kg per day. It is necessary that the diet should provide at least 150 kcal/kg per day to initiate recovery. In the past a great deal of emphasis was put on the amount of protein in the diet. It has now been realised that 2 g/kg body weight of protein is required for the regeneration of tissues, and amounts in excess of 3 g/kg/day are wasted and burnt as energy. Thus provision of adequate calories is more important than large amounts of protein. Carbohydrates in the form of sugar or starch will be bulky, and the best way of providing energy is in the form of fat, especially vegetable oil, which is better absorbed.

During convalescence, when appetite has returned, a child eating a balanced diet consumes 160 kcal/kg and 2–3 g protein/kg daily. The early days, however, are critical, as the child is desperately ill, the body's metabolic processes are at an ebb and additionally there may be complications like hypothermia, hypoglycaemia and infection. Moreover, anorexia and irritability make the feeding difficult. A liquid diet fed through a nasogastric tube is helpful at this stage and most clinicians find a milk-based formula, with the addition of casein and oil to increase the protein and calorie content, useful for initiating treatment. Originally, dried skim milk powder was used as the basis of the formula. It was fortified with casein, cottonseed oil and sucrose to provide the required protein and calories. Full-cream dried powdered milk has also been used in the same way. The various ingredients are mixed in proportions shown in Table 6.3. Potassium 1.0 g and magnesium 0.5 g are added to each 100 ml of the above diet to replenish tissue stores and to provide the

Table 6.3 *High energy–high protein formulae for initiating the treatment of PEM*

	Casein skim milk diet	Casein full-cream milk diet
Casein (g)	35	30
Dried skimmed milk (g)	35	–
Full cream milk (g)	–	60
Sugar (g)	35	30
Edible oil (g)	70	45
Water (ml)	1000	1000

requirements of the regenerating cells. The formula is administered at the rate of 110 ml/kg/day. Supplements of vitamin and iron are also necessary to make up the deficits and to provide the daily requirements.

As recovery occurs oedema is gradually lost – in a week or so – and appetite returns. At this stage solids can be introduced gradually until the child is able to take ordinary food.

Several complications need to be watched for. Of these the most important are hypothermia, hypoglycaemia and sepsis. Persistent hypothermia even with frequent feeding is a danger signal and is often due to underlying infection. Severe diarrhoea due to lactose intolerance occurs in a small number of cases and responds well to the removal of lactose from the child's diet. After a week or so on a lactose-free diet ordinary milk feeds can be tolerated, though in some cases lactose intolerance is known to persist for several weeks.

Careful control of electrolyte disturbances and infection, as well as rational dietary management, have helped to reduce the previously high rates of mortality. In most cases management is possible at the level of the health centre or the sub-centre without the need for complex laboratory support.

Hospital management

The trend hitherto has been to consider PEM as any acute disease and to treat it in hospital. More recently doubts have been raised with regard to the suitability of the hospital for treating all forms of malnutrition. The cost of hospital treatment is high. In countries where childhood malnutrition is common it is not unusual to find 20–40 per cent of hospital beds taken up by patients with malnutrition. Cross-infection in hospital is usual, and often a child recovers from malnutrition only to succumb to some infection. Hence case fatality for hospital treatment is high. Moreover, after all this investment in time, effort and cost, children are usually discharged to that same home environment where the disorder first started.

However, a case can be made for treating severe cases *initially* in hospital. These children are desperately ill; many of them are likely to develop complications and are in need of intensive care.

Home management

There is now a growing experience of the benefits of treating the child with mild to moderate malnutrition at home, within the family environment and the community. In several imaginative programmes successful use has been made of the health visitor and village health worker to achieve rehabilitation of such cases at home using locally available foods. The parents see their children improve with better feeding, and come to appreciate the importance of many of the locally available foods in the weaning of children. Moreover, the food is prepared utilising only the resources of the village home. Under supervision, the mother learns skills which will benefit other children in the family as well as the neighbourhood. This change of emphasis from the hospital ward to the home and family environment for the management of malnutrition has, in turn, led to several innovative approaches for dealing with the problem at the community level.

INNOVATIVE APPROACHES

Nutrition rehabilitation centres (Figures 6.6a and b)

The nutrition rehabilitation centre was first described in the 1960s as a convalescent place or staging post between the hospital ward and the home. Two advantages were immediately obvious. Firstly, it took the pressure off the crowded hospital wards where treatment costs were becoming prohibitive. Secondly, nutrition education of the mothers was easier to organise and more effective in the relatively quiet environment of the nutrition rehabilitation centre in comparison with the bustle in the acute paediatric ward. Soon the activities of the nutrition rehabilitation centre were expanded to include training in mothercraft, in improved techniques of farming, raising poultry, environmental sanitation and other similar activities. When the activities of the nutrition rehabilitation centres were integrated with those of the out-patient services and under-5s clinics, they became the focal points of maternal and

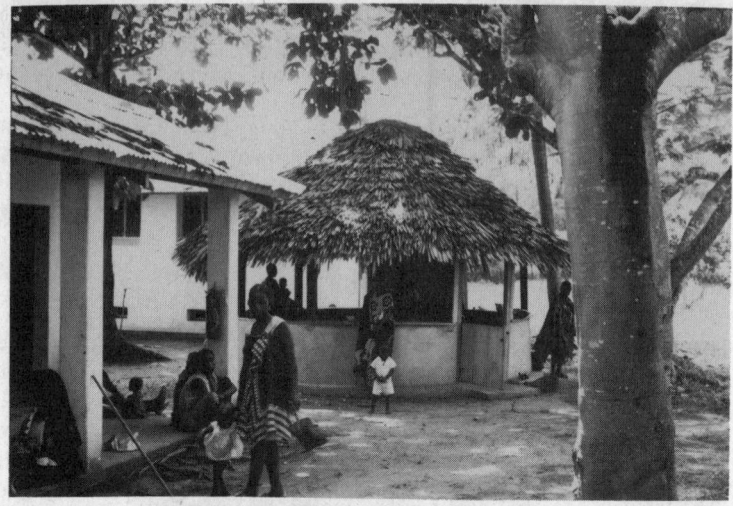

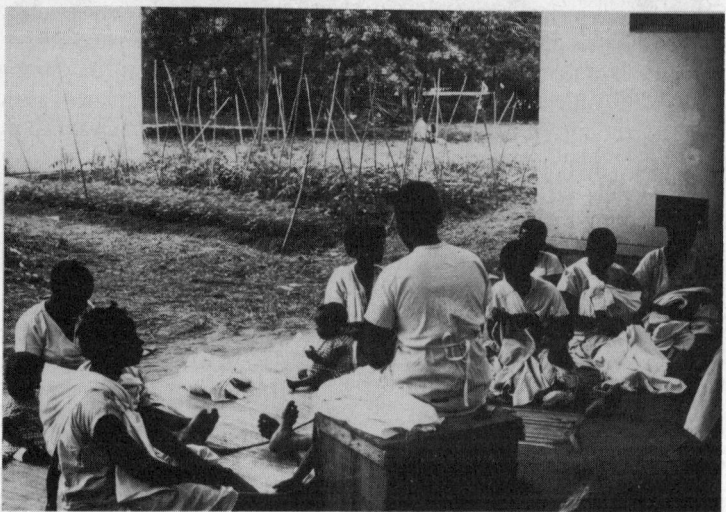

Figure 6.6 (a) Nutrition rehabilitation centre; (b) Mothers in discussion, with the vegetable plot in the background

child health work and of disseminating new knowledge in the community. Mothers admitted to such centres often take on the role of advisers in child feeding in their immediate neighbourhood. This has the advantage of creating a locally available source of knowledge in infant feeding for the community.

The nutrition rehabilitation centre is basically a school for parents who come together as either residents or day visitors to learn about better ways of feeding their children. They learn by participation and by observing their children thrive on foods which they have cooked at the centre. Thus, in leading the child back to health the emphasis has shifted from the hospital environment to the home environment. Health workers now step back and allow the auxiliaries to take over as educators and demonstrators. The emphasis is on locally available foods, prepared and cooked in the home kitchen, and as befits the domestic economy. The facilities consist of a residential unit or a ward with a kitchen and a plot of land where the foods used in the daily cooking are grown. The objective is to demonstrate the cooking of multimixes which provide adequate calories and protein in manageable bulk.

The development of the nutrition rehabilitation centres has been a useful step towards integration of treatment with prevention. After the initial period of acute illness, medical care is actively replaced by informed lay care as recovery proceeds. Moreover, there is cross-fertilisation between medicine and several other related disciplines like community development, agriculture, education and social sciences. Such a unified team approach gives better results than the individual activities of the same disciplines based on rigid departmental lines.

A recent evaluation in Uganda, Peru, Haiti and Guatemala has proved that children attending these centres *do* show improved growth and nutrition recuperation in an impressive way. The cost per child per day ranged from US$372 in Haiti to US$876 in Guatemala, and even though ten to forty times less than that of hospitalisation, can still be called excessive. The effect of the nutrition rehabilitation centre on the knowledge of the mother was not always impressive. Thus there is still a great deal of room for improvement.

COMMUNITY-CENTRED APPROACHES

Several shortcomings of the nutrition rehabilitation centre are obvious, even though it is a significant advance compared to the hospital ward for the treatment of malnutrition. Only a small proportion of all children suffering from malnutrition in the community are brought to a health facility for treatment, and only a proportion of these will be eventually admitted to the nutrition rehabilitation centre. Thus a centre can provide only limited coverage. It is physically impossible to provide one centre for each village in a country. Secondly, nutrition rehabilitation centres treat children after malnutrition has occurred. What most countries need is a preventive/promotive activity.

For these reasons, health workers have experimented with more community-centred approaches. For this purpose a new look at the problem of childhood malnutrition and our methods of dealing with it is necessary. Traditionally we tend to think of malnutrition as any other disease in which the problem is at the family level and the management is also aimed at the level of the patient and his family. But malnutrition is a problem at the level of the community, and is the consequence of the prevailing state of cultural, social and technical development. A community which is able to feed its children is in a healthier state of development compared to one which cannot. One must therefore search for solutions within the community on the principle that 'the state of nutrition is determined by what people do and not by what they get'. Amongst the community-based programmes are those for increasing productivity at the village level, preparation of weaning diets from local foods in the form of multimixes, child feeding programmes supported by community effort, identification of beneficiaries for community assistance by village health workers using simple techniques, and other similar activities. Many of these activities supplement the effects of services like the under-5s clinics described earlier, and together prepare the community for programmes of integrated development. Thus, in Hyderabad (India) the village community was mobilised to create farmers' groups who raised crops on communal plots; the women in turn processed these foods into a nourishing multimix, the village health workers identified children in need of food supplementation and all these activities were strongly supported by a network of community health activities. In Jamkhed (India) the community increases its agricultural potential by building earth dams across streams, and young farmers' clubs raise crops for a village feeding programme which is supervised by village health committees and operated by the village health workers.

These are some of the new approaches. But they are all in experimental stages and operating within defined boundaries. For them to spread both nationally and internationally a new breed of professional is needed who is capable of identifying the social, ecological and other root causes of nutritional disorders, and of working with the community to find solutions.

MONITORING THE NUTRITION OF THE COMMUNITY

The health worker usually operates from the district hospital or health centre, and the community to be served is defined administratively or by geographical boundaries. The first need is to get to know one's community well. It is important to obtain an ordnance map of the area and the latest census data. Other government departments like agriculture, community development, water supply, education and so on may have useful information about the area and the people. A study of annual reports of these departments supplemented with reports of any surveys carried out can provide information on land availability, agricultural productivity, literacy, rates, employment, local industry as well as local beliefs and practices. Meetings and discussions with local leaders and officials may also help to add further details about the community and its problems. The best source of information, however, can come through familiarising oneself with the area and its people during community rounds.

Is malnutrition a problem in the community? Hospital admission figures and out-patient registers provide a useful clue to its presence in the community. When malnutrition is being commonly diagnosed in the health institutions it is important that the extent of the problem be measured in the community, always bearing in mind that most health institutions mainly serve the community in their immediate neighbourhood. Many cases of malnutrition, and especially the mild-moderate forms, may not be brought to the notice of the health workers, and hence it is useful to measure their prevalence in the community.

All health workers are not in the fortunate position of having the resources to carry out extensive surveys, but this should not prevent them from measuring the effectiveness of their activities at regular intervals. Several techniques of rapid rural assessment have been described recently and can be used to advantage by health workers in isolated rural areas with poor facilities and support.

MAKING A COMMUNITY DIAGNOSIS OF MALNUTRITION

Depending upon the resources available, weight-for-age, height-for-age, arm circumference and arm circumference-for-height (Quac Stick) may be used as parameters for measuring the growth and the nutritional status of children. Clearly it is not possible to measure all the children in the area and it may only be possible to measure the children in one or two villages at a time. However, if these villages are selected with forethought, a useful picture of the whole district can be put together over a couple of years. Many villages have a population of about 1000 persons, and often villages and hamlets are in clusters. The desirable minimum for statistical purposes is about 50 children under the age of 3 years per village. For truly useful information about the dietary pattern, the recommended number is 300 children under the age of 3 years. Depending upon the size of the village or of the residential area (e.g. squatter settlement), the number of households to be visited is indicated in Table 6.4. The information obtained through such surveys can be aug-

Table 6.4 *Number of children to be included in a survey of households for assessing nutrition*

No. of people in the settlement	No. of children in the settlement	No. of children for measuring	No. of houses in the settlement	Homes to visit
100	20	20	5-7	All houses
500	100	100	25-30	All houses
1000	200	200	50-70	All houses
2000	400	200	50-70	Every 2nd house
5000	1000	200	50-70	Every 5th house

mented through lay reporting. Various members of the community, such as village health workers, school teachers, or school children can gather information using the arm band and/or the Quac Stick, as well as a simple questionnaire on infant feeding. In the case of the latter, as well as in general discussions with community leaders, it is useful to follow four areas of enquiry, *viz.*:

(1) What do informants say people ought to do? (Assesses level of knowledge).
(2) What do informants say most people do? (Provides a measure of beliefs and practices).
(3) What do informants say they themselves do? (Gives a measure of common dietary patterns).
(4) What do informants and others actually do? (This information is obtained through actual observations and recall type of enquiry).

The traditional birth attendants in the community are usually knowledgeable and can provide valuable information on family life patterns, dietary practices and attitudes, details of pregnancies as well as birth weights and birth intervals.

When all the information discussed above is assembled, it is possible to construct a nutrition profile of the community. The proportion of infants with low birth weight, percentage low weight for age, percentage with low arm circumference, percentage with low arm circumference for height, percentage low weight for height, birth intervals, high-risk pregnancies, family stability, customs and taboos, use of fats and oils in the dietaries and similar other information can be obtained about life patterns in the different settlements and communities of the district. Malnutrition is common in communities who do not receive adequate health and other services. Hence indicators of health coverage provide useful contributory information. Availability and acceptance of prenatal care, attendance at the under-5s clinics as judged by the presence of a weight chart at home and the regularity of weighing, coverage by immunisation, local facilities for oral rehydration to treat diarrhoea and acceptance of family planning services serve as measures of the quality of health coverage of the community. Malnutrition is also the consequence of the prevailing state of cultural, social and technical development of the community as well as the sharing of resources. Hence socio-economic indicators such as availability of safe water in adequate amounts, facilities for disposal of human waste, literacy rates, employment or availability of land, type of dwellings and so on help to assess the determinants of malnutrition in the community.

Malnutrition is considered to be prevalent when results of community surveys show the following:

(1) the number of children with marasmus and those with oedema is greater than 20 per cent;
(2) the number of children with severe anaemia is greater than 5 per cent;
(3) the number of children under-weight exceeds 20 per cent;
(4) the number of children dying is greater than 20 per cent of total children born to mothers in the community.

Alleviation and eradication of hunger requires community action. Hence community awareness and interest are important. The sharing of all information with the community helps to create rapport and exchange of ideas. Several of the community programmes mentioned in the preceding section have active community participation as the primary objective. In the sharing of information and exchange of ideas one may discover the beginnings of community-based interventions.

In all surveys and activities for monitoring the impact of services it is important to be aware of certain pitfalls. Those who are in greatest need are usually out of sight. It is the remote village away from the main road where the need is most acute. It is the disadvantaged in the community, such as for example, the lower castes or the single-parent families, whose voice is rarely heard in the dialogue with the community. Subjects like low wages, often below the statutory minimum wage, the iron grip of the big landlords, high interest rates and consequent indebtedness, and unemployment rarely get discussed in the open and need to be looked for. Interviews with the disadvantaged in small groups may provide useful information. The effects of the seasons must also be taken into account. If one has established a regular pattern of community or village rounds, then visiting the same place just before and soon after the wet season may provide useful insights. Finally, all surveys are snapshots and not trends. Hence one should be careful about drawing firm conclusions and making generalisations.

The objective of monitoring services and programmes is to bring about improvements in their effectiveness and efficiency. Technical innovations, policy decisions and administrative changes are all part of the process. A question often asked is, 'How can health and nutrition interventions alter destitution and poverty? Surely political decisions and socioeconomic development are the answers!' This is true to a large extent, but health workers can contribute a great deal by slanting the services to seek out and help the neediest. Health services, like other national programmes in most countries, are largely monopolised by the elite. To be able to identify those at greatest risk and ensure their health and welfare will be one way to alleviate poverty; for to ensure freedom from illness and incapacity is to ensure availability for employment. To create self-sufficiency through locally available foods is to save scarce family resources. Community cohesion will ensure community support for the disadvantaged. To help promote functional literacy is to enable the disadvantaged to fend for themselves in a hostile world. Health and nutrition interventions hold the promise of becoming springboards for community upliftment.

FURTHER READING

Alleyne, G. A. O., Hay, R. W., Picou, D. I., Stanfield, J. P. and Whitehead, R. G. *Protein-energy Malnutrition*. Edward Arnold, London, 1977.

Coward, W. A. and Lunn, P. G. The biochemistry and physiology of kwashiorkor and marasmus. *Br. Med. Bull*. (1981), **37**, 25-30.

Gopalan, C. Kwashiorkor and marasmus. Evolution and distinguishing features. In McCance, R. A. and Widdowson, E. M. (eds) *Calorie Deficiency and Protein Deficiency*. J. & A. Churchill, London, 1968.

Morley, D. and Woodland, M. *See How they Grow – monitoring child growth for appropriate health care in developing countries*. Macmillan, Basingstoke and London, 1979.

Olson, P.E. (ed.) *Protein-calorie Malnutrition*. Academic Press, New York and London, 1975.

Shakir, A. The surveillance of protein-calorie malnutrition by simple and economical means – a report to UNICEF. *J. Trop. Ped*. (1975), **21**, 69-85.

World Health Organization: Rapid village nutrition survey technique. WHO Regional Office for Africa AFR/NUT/84. Brazzaville, 1977 (mimeo.)

World Health Organization. *A growth chart for international use in maternal and child health care.* Guidelines for primary health care personnel. WHO, Geneva, 1978.

Chapter 7

Vitamins in Health and Disease

VITAMIN A AND XEROPHTHALMIA

Xerophthalmia and its most serious manifestation, keratomalacia, have probably occurred in badly fed communities throughout human history. The condition was well known to Hippocrates who described the use of liver in its treatment. Throughout the nineteenth century a number of papers describing xerophthalmia had been published from different parts of the world, including during the Irish potato famine in 1848. An important observation was made during the First World War in Denmark which helped to associate deficiency of vitamin A with xerophthalmia. Butter was replaced by margarine in the Danish diet during this war and defatted milk was commonly used for infant feeding, with the result that there was an outbreak of xerophthalmia and keratomalacia amongst Danish children. Amongst the affected children the fatality rate at the time was 24 per cent. Several reports from Indonesia have quoted fatality rates of 35 per cent. Partly because xerophthalmia indicates a severe form of nutritional disorder, and partly because the visually handicapped child finds it difficult to fend for himself in the harsh environment of the tropics, severe xerophthalmia invariably carries a poor prognosis. In Surabaya a follow-up study of discharged severe xerophthalmia cases revealed that 40 per cent of the children had died within a few years. More recently in Hyderabad, India, it has been reported that 30 per cent of the children with keratomalacia had died within 3-4 months after discharge from hospital. Generally speaking, 25 per cent of the survivors of severe xerophthalmia with keratomalacia remain totally blind, about 50-60 per cent become partially blind and only 15-20 per cent escape with unimpaired sight. These figures indicate the seriousness of the condition.

The size of the problem on a global scale was not fully appreciated until 1962 when a survey sponsored by WHO showed vitamin A deficiency to be a major cause of blindness in children in all the 30 countries in South East Asia, Africa and Latin America included in this survey.

It was then estimated that every year 85 000 cases of blindness occurred in children due to xerophthalmia, chiefly in the rice-eating countries of South East Asia. Recently, a prospective longitudinal field study involving 4600 pre-school children was carried out in rural Java over a period of 2 years. The incidence of corneal xerophthalmia was 5 per 1000/year. A randomised multistage cluster survey of 27 084 rural children in Indonesia showed that the prevalence of active corneal disease in pre-school children was 6.4 per 10 000. By extrapolation of these findings the authors estimate that every year 500 000 new cases of xerophthalmia occur in the four South East Asian countries of India, Bangladesh, Indonesia and the Philippines. Half of these cases lead to loss of sight, with an eventual high mortality. In India, several nutrition surveys suggest that 8–10 per cent of rural children between 6 months and 6 years have signs of vitamin A deficiency, and of the country's estimated blind population of 4.5 million, about a quarter or a third owe their disability to the after-effects of vitamin A deficiency. The present estimates indicate that among the 92 million children aged 1–5 years in India, 7.4 million have non-corneal and 0.22 million suffer from corneal xerophthalmia at any given time. Out of these arise the annual numbers of 52 000 blind and between 110 000 and 132 000 partially blind. In Bangladesh, it is estimated that at least 17 000 children between the ages of 0 and 6 years lose their sight each year on account of xerophthalmia. A nutrition survey in Jordan showed blood levels of vitamin A within the 'deficit' range ($<$10 μg/100 ml) in 5 per cent and 'low' (10–20 μg/100 ml) in a further 39 per cent of the children examined. Thus, clinical vitamin A deficiency represents only the tip of the iceberg. There are many more amongst the apparently healthy community with poor body stores who can be precipitated into an acute deficiency state.

Many children with clinical vitamin A deficiency have advanced eye lesions when first seen. This may be due to the rapid progress of lesions once they are established, or because of difficulties in access to medical facilities. In Central Java, out of 8000 cases of xerophthalmia seen in 1960 in an eye clinic, 8 per cent had advanced lesions likely to cause loss of vision, and twice this number had moderate lesions which were expected to respond to treatment, but leaving residual corneal scarring. Furthermore, not all those blinded by xerophthalmia survive. Deficiency of vitamin A is commonly associated with protein-calorie malnutrition and other nutritional deficiencies. The common observation is that for every survivor from advanced xerophthalmia there is another who dies.

Epidemiology

The peak prevalence of xerophthalmia is in the third and fourth years of life. In this respect it differs from PEM, which has its highest frequency at the age of 18 months. It is a condition seen almost always in a growing child. Depletion of body stores takes much longer in adults, since growth has ceased and utilisation of vitamin A for the growth of new cells is much less.

In the search for a specific dietary cause of xerophthalmia it is often forgotten that vitamin A deficiency is a social disease affecting the poorest sections of the community who are forced to live on a monotonous diet and suffer recurrent illnesses. Socioeconomic development in many countries has resulted in a fall in the incidence of xerophthalmia and the condition is now rare in Hong Kong, Singapore and Taiwan, and the Middle East where it used to be common. Social upheavals, on the other hand, cause widespread hardships and precipitate xerophthalmia and other deficiency disorders, as happened in Bangladesh and South Vietnam.

Vitamin A deficiency is especially common in the rice-eating areas of South East Asia where 2-8 per cent of all pre-school children may show clinical manifestations. The wheat-eating countries of West Asia and North Africa have fewer cases. In tropical Africa, on the other hand, xerophthalmia is not common and only a few cases are seen, usually in association with long-standing PEM. In West Africa the common use of red palm oil in cooking acts as a major protective measure against vitamin A deficiency.

The primary cause of low body stores of vitamin A is dietary deficiency caused by a monotonous diet made up almost entirely of rice. Protective foods with high β-carotene content like amaranth, carrots, spinach and paw-paw are not offered because of local traditions and beliefs that such foods give rise to diarrhoea in children or because of ignorance. The result is a low intake of vitamin A or its precursor. Dietary surveys in several rural communities in South East Asia show that the average daily intake of vitamin A in children is 70 μg compared to the requirement of 300 μg. By comparison the average daily intake in affluent western communities is 1200-3000 μg. Such low intakes condition a community to xerophthalmia, and acute deficiency of vitamin A then occurs amongst those sections of the community who suffer a high prevalence of precipitating factors like infective illness, lack of personal hygiene and poor environmental conditions. Such a conceptual framework to explain the aetiology of xerophthalmia is essential for mounting successful programmes of prevention. Thus, even though the disease presents itself as an acute deficiency of vitamin A, this deficiency occurs on a background of recurrent infections, poverty, lack of hygiene, non-availability of health care, inadequate food and general underdevelopment.

Some children with such a background of deficient intake combined with poor living conditions may progress to show clinical signs of xerophthalmia or Bitot's spots (shiny, grey triangular spots on the conjunctiva) either alone or in combination with protein-calorie malnutrition. A history of night-blindness is a useful screening tool. It has been shown to correlate closely with other evidence of vitamin A deficiency. More commonly an intercurrent illness leads to a sudden loss of vitamin A from the body followed by acute onset of clinical disease. Several disease processes are known to cause a loss of vitamin A from the body. In tuberculosis, pneumonia, urinary tract infections and other chronic diseases, massive excretion of the vitamin in the urine has been recorded. For example, in adult patients suffering from pneumonia such a loss has been estimated to be in the range of 1000 μg/day. Common childhood infections such as diarrhoea, upper respiratory infections, bronchitis and chicken pox have been shown to cause a fall in plasma vitamin A levels of between 10 and 30 μg/dl. In children, measles, whooping cough and recurrent diarrhoea are common precipitating factors. Seasonal epidemics of these illnesses in rural communities leave in their wake many children with acute vitamin A deficiency. A variety of infections can impair absorption of vitamin A. For example, malabsorption has been demonstrated in acute diarrhoea, ascariasis, giardiasis, severe hookworm infestations as well as in salmonella infections and in schistosomiasis.

It is not widely known that ocular pathology can progress rapidly. A child brought to an out-patient clinic with Bitot's spots and some corneal involvement can deteriorate within a day and develop keratomalacia progressing to total destruction of the cornea unless vitamin A is administered in adequate doses and immediate steps are taken to protect the eye and to correct coexisting nutritional deficiencies, (figure 7.1).

Seasonal variations in prevalence rates have been reported from many countries. These variations are not always explained by changes in intake. Possibly they are related to seasonal variations in growth or in the seasonal incidence of intercurrent illnesses. In most countries where xerophthalmia is endemic there is a summer peak in incidence rates following diarrhoeal illnesses and a winter peak coinciding with respiratory infections.

Physiology of vitamin A

Vitamin A is obtained in the diet either as preformed vitamin A or as β-carotene. In the average western diet half of the vitamin A activity is provided as carotene and the other half as preformed vitamin A. In the peasant communities of the developing world β-carotene is the major

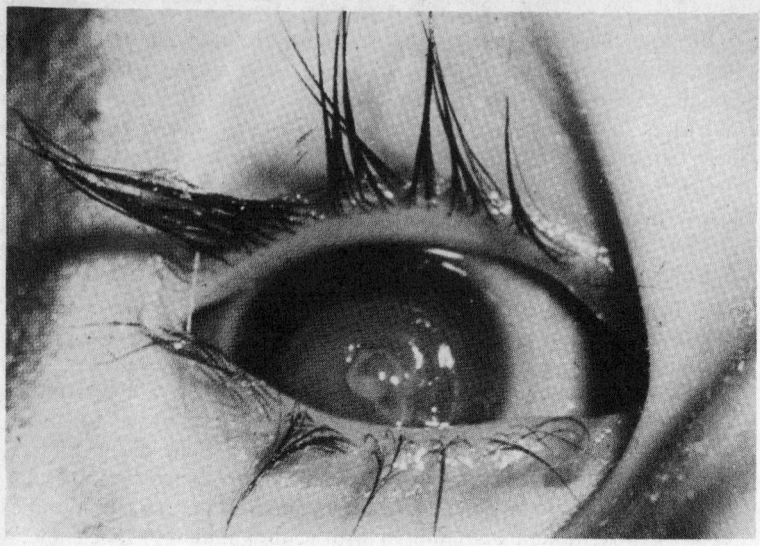

Figure 7.1   Destruction of the cornea in blinding malnutrition

source of the vitamin. The cells of the intestinal mucosa convert β-carotene to vitamin A. Two molecules of β-carotene give rise to one of retinol, though the theoretical yield is hardly ever reached and, in general, the activity of β-carotene is about a sixth of vitamin A.

Preformed vitamin A occurs in food in the form of long-chain retinyl esters. These are hydrolysed in the intestinal lumen by means of pancreatic hydrolase and also by a similar enzyme present on the brush border. Within the mucosal cells the retinol is rapidly re-esterified and later transported in the lymphatics within chylomicrons. Under normal conditions over 90 per cent of ingested vitamin A is absorbed. When it reaches the vascular compartment the retinyl esters are removed from the circulation almost entirely by the liver, and stored in the liver cells as fat globules. When required, vitamin A is mobilised from the liver cells and carried bound to a specific transport protein – the retinol binding protein (RBP). In the circulation, RBP occurs in combination with pre-albumin in the form of a protein-protein complex. In protein deficiency states the release of vitamin A from hepatic stores is affected because of defective hepatic production of carrier proteins including RBP. It is likely that the low levels of vitamin A in PEM reflect a functional impairment in hepatic release of vitamin A rather than vitamin deficiency as such, for the hepatic release of the vitamin is improved with adequate feeding without supplementary vitamin A.

β-carotene is solubilised less well in the gut lumen. Under normal conditions about 70 per cent of β-carotene is absorbed. It is then converted to retinaldehyde in the cells of the intestinal mucosa, followed by reduction to retinol and esterification. The ester is then incorporated into chylomicra and transported via the lymphatics and finally taken up by the liver.

The provitamin A activity of different carotenoids varies considerably. Up to now it has been customary to assume that 1 μg of retinol is equivalent to 6 μg of β-carotene and 12 μg of mixed dietary carotenoids.

The role of vitamin A in the production of visual purple and for the integrity of the conjunctival and corneal epithelium is well established. Almost all the clinical signs of vitamin A deficiency are related to vision and the eye, *viz.* night-blindness, dryness of conjunctiva, Bitot's spots, keratomalacia with scarring and destruction of the cornea resulting in blindness (figure 7.1). However, there is no way of identifying what cases of conjunctival xerosis or Bitot's spot are associated with *active* vitamin A deficiency, except by observing their response to therapy. Involvement of more than the temporal quadrant of the conjunctiva, presence of night-blindness and of punctate keratopathy are important clues to the presence of active deficiency; but the sensitivity of these clues is only 50–80 per cent. A sizeable proportion of active cases do not have xerosis outside the temporal quadrants. History of night-blindness may not be forthcoming and diagnosis of punctate keratopathy requires a slit lamp. But when these signs occur in pre-school children urgent treatment with vitamin A is indicated.

Recent work in laboratory animals indicates that vitamin A is necessary for growth; in fact measurement of growth has been used as an assay for vitamin A activity in the rat. Abnormalities in RNA metabolism and protein synthesis do occur in severe vitamin A deficiency, but do not cause striking clinical signs as in the case of xerophthalmia.

Approaches to prevention

Clinical vitamin A deficiency needs urgent treatment because of the tendency for rapid deterioration in the eye. Vitamin A is necessary especially when there are obvious signs of PEM and if ocular lesions are advanced. Parenteral administration is also necessary if there is associated diarrhoea and vomiting and where oral administration cannot be relied upon. In such cases intramuscular injection of the water-miscible form 100 000 i.u. should be administered on diagnosis, followed by 100 000 i.u. of the oily preparation by mouth on the following day and another 100 000–200 000 i.u. of oil preparation orally prior to discharge. In several studies of severe xerophthalmia oral administration of oil-miscible preparation in a dose of 200 000 i.u. has been found as effective as 100 000 i.u. of water-miscible preparation given intramuscularly. On the other hand, intramuscular administration of oily vitamin A is not effective and such preparations are best avoided.

There is clearly a need for health and nutrition education in all developing countries, but this is a slow process and urgent solutions are necessary. This is more so because blindness due to xerophthalmia is preventable. Amongst the various approaches developed the nutrition rehabilitation centre and mass prophylaxis with vitamin A are the most promising. The nutrition rehabilitation centre was described in the previous chapter and is best suited for rehabilitation of children suffering from xerophthalmia complicated by PEM. Parents of children who have been admitted to such a centre become useful sources of knowledge on child feeding in their neighbourhood. Moreover, the centre itself provides opportunities for the training of village health workers and auxiliaries. The first nutrition rehabilitation centre established in 1970 to deal with xerophthalmia in South India has been successful and has become the springboard of a large community programme.

In the last few years an imaginative approach has been tried out in several countries for the prevention of xerophthalmia. This approach is based on the fact that vitamin A is a depot vitamin and it should therefore be possible to fill the depot. After several field trials it has been found that a dose of 200 000 i.u. of vitamin A in oil given orally is tolerated well. When administered every 6 months such a dose is able to maintain adequate tissue stores and protects against xerophthalmia. Laboratory studies with labelled vitamin A have shown that about 47 per cent of the orally administered dose in oil is retained in the body. Observations in communities with well-developed programmes of mass prophylaxis have shown a significant fall in the incidence of ocular manifestations of vitamin A deficiency. Several countries have now adopted this method for the prevention of childhood blindness.

The above interventions no doubt are major advances and open the way to dealing with this tragic problem. However, by themselves they are not enough. Blinding malnutrition is a marker of the most severe form of deprivation. Even though it presents as a deficiency disease, the contributory factors are undernourishment added to infective illness and lack of adequate care. There is now a growing awareness that in the urban shanty towns and squatter settlements the incidence may be higher, especially when the mother has to go out to work leaving the care of the infant to an older sib. The problem is made more acute as breast feeding is being replaced by over-dilute milk formula or feeding with condensed milk. In such a situation, periodic dosing with vitamin A can be no better than papering over the cracks. Appropriate programmes of primary care providing basic health services and health education together with protection from common infectious illnesses of childhood are the obvious needs of such communities. Within such programmes of regular health surveillance periodic dosing with vitamin A could have a maximum impact. Xerophthalmia is the burden of neglected communities. Its eradication lies in the provision of regular health care together with the availability of vitamin A in a balanced diet.

RICKETS AND METABOLIC BONE DISEASE

Rickets is primarily a disease of children in the first 2 years of life when rapid skeletal growth causes increased requirements of vitamin D and minerals. It is a disease of calcium and phosphorus metabolism which occurs when infants and children receive insufficient vitamin D.

The clinical effects of vitamin D deficiency are mainly seen in the growing parts of the bone, the epiphyses of long bones (figure 7.2) and the costochondral junctions. In addition the bones of the body become soft due to poor mineralisation and deformities like bow-legs occur on weight-bearing. In the active stage of rickets the child looks ill. He is pale, irritable, sleepless and at times may suffer from tetany and convulsions. But the disease is very rarely fatal in itself, except that respiratory infections tend to be more frequent in rickets. The most important effects of the disease are retarded physical growth and skeletal deformities due to a disorder of bone calcification.

Epidemiology

HISTORICAL

Rickets was known in ancient times and it is most likely that sporadic cases occurred in the larger cities throughout the Middle Ages. The first full description of the disease was written in the seventeenth century by the English physician Glisson. Throughout the eighteenth and first half of the nineteenth century rickets was common in the cities of western and central Europe. It reached its peak prevalence in the latter half of the nineteenth century and in the first decade of the present century. The rise of textile industries in England led to the employment of women and children, and to crowded living conditions in the cities. As slums grew, sunlight became scarcer in the lives of many of the working population. This, added to the unhygienic methods of child-rearing such as swaddling and being kept indoors without opportunity for outdoor play, led to a great rise in the incidence of rickets. In industrial cities of Britain the disease was almost universal and came to

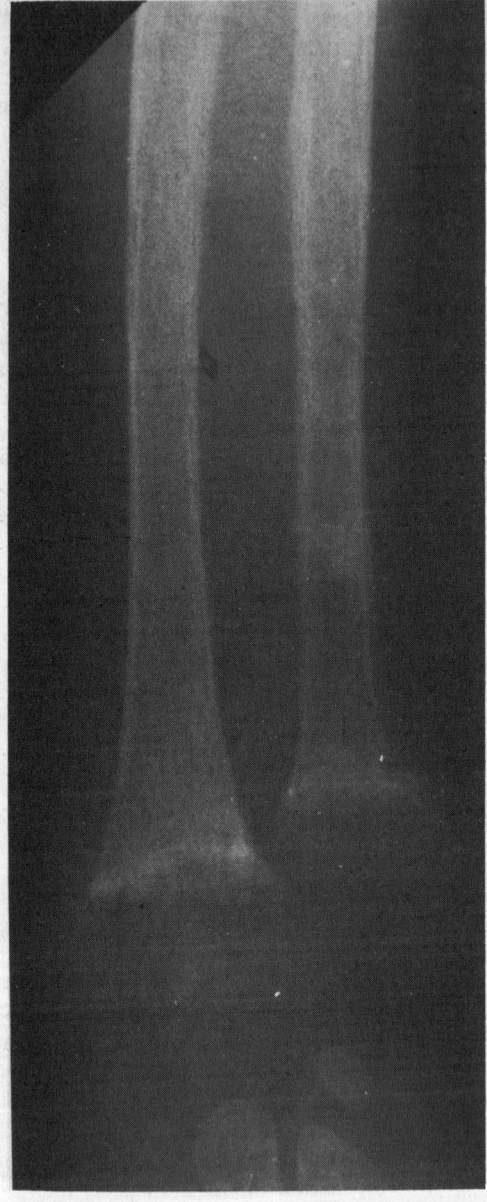

Figure 7.2 X-ray of the wrist, showing abnormalities in the growing ends of the radius and ulna. Note the fraying and cupping of the epiphyseal end with poor calcification

be known as the 'English disease', even though it was equally common elsewhere. In 1907, in the hospitals of Paris one of every two children between 6 months and 3 years of age showed evidence of rickets. In Boston it was estimated that 80 per cent of the children of poorer classes suffered from the disease. In 1921 it was estimated that fully three-quarters of the children in large cities like New York showed some evidence of rickets. At about the same time a third of infants born in Glasgow were said to suffer from it.

When the beneficial effects of sunlight and cod liver oil were recognised it became possible to bring rickets under control, and the disease has now been virtually eliminated from many of the larger cities of industrial nations. In Britain the principal early measure against rickets was cod liver oil, issued through the infant welfare clinics. Throughout the 1920s and the 1930s, the use of cod liver oil was promoted by the infant welfare services, with the result that at the outbreak of the Second World War rickets had become a rare disease in Britain. About this time further nutritional measures were introduced in the form of a free supply of cod liver oil and vitamin D for infants and pregnant mothers, fortification of infant foods with vitamin D, enrichment of margarine with vitamins A and D, and addition of calcium carbonate to wheat flour. As a result of these measures rickets became rare towards the end of the war.

RESURGENCE OF RICKETS IN RECENT YEARS

In the early 1960s rickets reappeared in Britain. This time it was mainly confined to immigrants from the Indian subcontinent and the West Indies. An incidence of 30 per cent overt rickets and osteomalacia in children and adult women has been reported in some studies. If abnormal biochemical findings are also included, the prevalence of vitamin D deficiency rises to 74 per cent in children and 53 per cent in adults. Several studies of the dietary habits of immigrant groups show that there is a prompt abandonment of breast feeding even though in the homeland the baby not breast-fed has little chance of survival. In contrast, the adult feeding habits remain virtually unchanged.

In spite of these different dietary habits, the nutrient content of the diet of the immigrant child, including the intake of vitamin D, was not different from that of a control group of Scottish children. There is also no significant difference in the diets of rachitic and non-rachitic immigrant children. It would therefore seem that the non-dietary source of vitamin D is important. These observations are borne out by studies of vitamin D status in immigrant groups in comparison with that of communities in their countries of origin. Such studies show that, despite the similarity in diets, Asians in Britain have a higher incidence of biochemical abormalities suggestive of rickets than similar groups in the homeland. Exposure to sunlight is thus an important aetiological factor in vitamin D deficiency. Women and children amongst the immigrant groups are more at risk because of staying indoors and, especially in the former, the traditional way of dressing which exposes few body parts to sunlight.

Rickets in the tropics and subtropics

In many countries of sub-Saharan Africa rickets is rare. As the cities grow and industry develops it is likely that many of these countries will experience a rising incidence of rickets.

In India, a frequency of 0.9 per cent in urban and 1.5 per cent in rural children of low socioeconomic groups has been reported. Again the sprawling slums of the large cities in Asia and Latin America are likely to be the major factors in the incidence of rickets. Osteomalacia in women, on the other hand, is relatively common. In New Delhi, one hospital has reported admitting 60 patients with advanced osteomalacia per year. In the majority the presenting signs are those of vague pain in the back and legs, but in about 10 per cent tetany is the first symptom. Most are women in the reproductive period and in many of them repeated pregnancies are contributory factors.

Rickets is relatively more common in the Middle East where women observe the Muslim tradition of 'purdah' and parents are reluctant to expose children to the burning sun. In a survey in four countries of North Africa (Morocco, Algeria, Tunisia, Libya), sponsored by WHO in 1965, rickets was noted in 10-11 per cent of children admitted to hospital or attending out-patient clinics in Morocco and Algeria. In Tunisia and Libya the frequency was 3 and 5 per cent respectively in similar groups of children.

Physiological mechanisms

Very few natural foods provide vitamin D (table 7.1), with the exception of fish. Fish liver oils have traditionally been major sources of the vitamin, before a synthetic vitamin became widely available. Fish obtain their vitamin D from eating plankton exposed to sunlight on the surface of the sea.

Many people obtain no vitamin D from the diet and their entire source of the vitamin is from the skin through exposure to sunlight. The average British diet provides 2.7 μg of vitamin D per day compared to the daily requirements of 10 μg. Of this amount in the diet, about a

Table 7.1 Sources of vitamin D (recommended intake 10 µg (400 i.u.))

Food	Range (µg/100 g)
Fish	5-45
Egg (whole)	1.25-1.5
Egg (yolk)	4-10
Margarine (vitaminised)	2-9
Butter	0.25-2.5
Cheese	About 0.3
Milk	0.1
Cereals, vegetables and fruit	No vitamin D
Meat and white fish	Insignificant amounts

third comes from margarine enriched with the vitamin. Fish and eggs together provide another third and the remainder is obtained from milk and milk products. Thus, for the average Briton, exposure to sunlight provides twice as much vitamin as that in the diet. It has been estimated that the cheeks of a European infant (area 20 cm^2) can synthesise daily about 10 µg of vitamin D if adequately exposed to sunlight – sufficient protection against rickets.

7-dehydrocholesterol is the precursor of vitamin D in the skin. On exposure to the ultraviolet rays in sunlight (wavelength range 250-310 nm) it is converted to cholecalciferol (vitamin D_3). The exact mechanism by which it is absorbed from the skin is not known. As we have noted, dietary sources are only required when a person is shielded from effective sunlight by clothing, housing conditions or smog.

On absorption from the skin or the gut, vitamin D accumulates rapidly in the liver where it undergoes hydroxylation yielding 25-OH-D_3, which is the major circulating metabolite of the vitamin. Further hydroxylation occurs in the kidney giving rise to 1-25-$(OH)_2$-D_3 which is the active form of vitamin D and behaves like a calcium- and phosphate-mobilising hormone in the body. On account of its steroidal structure and because it behaves in the same manner as other steroidal hormones 1-25-$(OH)_2$-D_3 is now classified as a renal hormone. A specific binding protein in the plasma serves to carry the active compound in aqueous solution and delivers it to tissue cells.

Dietary and serum calcium levels play an important role in regulating the production of 1-25-$(OH)_2$-D_3 by the kidney. Low intake of calcium, causing low serum levels, stimulates the production of 1-25-$(OH)_2$-D_3 whereas diets high in calcium, leading to increased serum calcium concentration, suppress the production of 1-25-$(OH)_2$-D_3. Instead, there is a production of another metabolite, 24, 25-(OH)$_2$-D$_3$. Thus, at normal serum calcium levels the kidney produces both 1-25-(OH)$_2$-D$_3$ and 24, 25-(OH)$_2$-D$_3$. In hypocalcaemia there is preferential production of 1-25-(OH)$_2$-D$_3$ and in hypercalcaemia of 24, 25-(OH)$_2$-D$_3$. This effect is mediated through the parathyroid hormone. Low serum calcium levels stimulate parathyroid hormone secretion which, in turn, increases the production of 1-25-(OH)$_2$-D$_3$ by the kidney (figure 7.3).

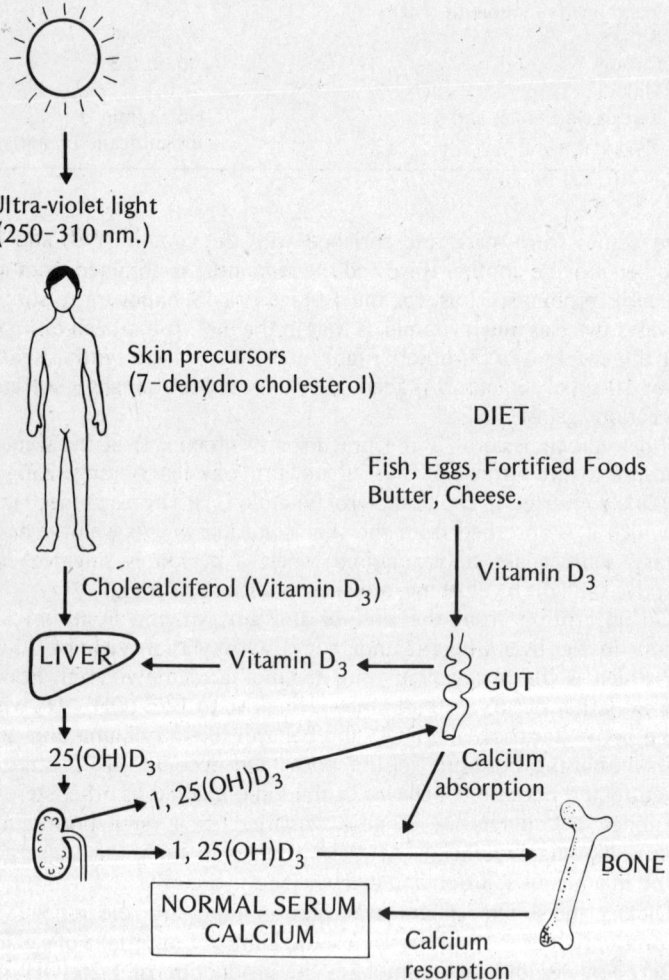

Figure 7.3   Physiology of vitamin D

The above observations are borne out by experiments in human volunteers. After the administration of oral vitamin D there is a delay of 16-20 hours before increased calcium uptake occurs. The time lag can be reduced to 6 hours by giving 25-OH-D_3, but the time lag still occurs indicating that it is 1-25-$(OH)_2$-D_3 which is the active compound. Under its influence calcium is absorbed from the gut and transported across mucosal cells in association with calcium-binding protein. A number of changes have been found in the brush border of the enterocyte in response to 1-25-$(OH)_2 D_3$. These include increased activities of alkaline phosphatase, increased synthesis of a number of proteins and other metabolic changes. The absorbed calcium then reaches the osteoid seams and growing cartilage of bone where it is incorporated.

In deficiency of vitamin D the growth zone of the epiphyseal cartilage is greatly enlarged and osteoid tissue accumulates on bony trabeculae where normally ossification would be taking place. It is difficult to define the effects of vitamin D on bone formation in simple terms of deposition and resorption. Instead the effect is one of endocrine synchronisation in the complex events of bone formation and turnover.

The kidney is also now recognised as a target organ for vitamin D activity besides being the site of formation of 1-25-$(OH)_2$-D_3. The effect is one of increased tubular reabsorption of phosphate, and to a lesser extent that of calcium and sodium. The renal response to the metabolites of Vitamin D is a part of phosphate homeostasis.

Calcium intake

With intakes below 600 mg per day most individuals are in negative calcium balance. On a dietary intake of 600-1000 mg a normal adult absorbs about half the ingested calcium and the net absorption varies little over this range. When calcium intakes fall below 500 mg adaptive mechanisms increase the proportion which is absorbed. In severe calcium restriction the efficiency of absorption can reach up to 70-80 per cent, mediated through increased production of 1-25-$(OH)_2$-D_3.

The daily intake of calcium in the diet and its source (table 7.2) vary from one population group to another and also from one individual to another depending upon dietary habits. In a global survey of calcium intake it was found that there were four broad groups of countries as follows:—

(1) Most of Europe and North America. The average intake of calcium is 900 mg/head/day. Of this 70-90 per cent is derived from milk and its products.
(2) Southern Europe and central South America. The average intake is

650–800 mg/head/day. Of this 50–70 per cent is from milk and milk products, but vegetables also make an important contribution.
(3) Chile, India, South Africa, Turkey, Egypt. The average intake is 350–500 mg/head/day. Of this, milk supplies 30–65 per cent, but cereals, pulses, vegetables and nuts also make a contribution.
(4) Japan. Intake is 350 mg or less derived fairly evenly from cereals, pulses, nuts, vegetables.

Table 7.2 *Calcium content of some common foods*

Food	Range (mg/100 g or 100 ml)
Milk – cow's fresh whole	120
Cheese – from whole or skimmed milk	80–1200
Eggs – fresh, white	50–60
Beef, mutton, pork and poultry	3–24
Pulses – raw dried	40–200
Vegetables – raw green leafy	25–250
Whole wheat – full extraction	30–40
Wheat flour – 70% extraction	13–20
Rice – raw polished	4–10
Maize	5–18
Millet	20–50
Potatoes – raw	7–10

Osteomalacia

This is characteristically found in women who live on cereal diets lacking in calcium and, for one reason or another, are mainly confined indoors. When they go out they are covered with clothing which prevents adequate exposure to sunlight. The most striking accounts have come from Northern India, North Africa and the Middle East where the condition is encountered in its more severe forms. More recently cases have been described from amongst immigrant Asian women in Britain. Symptoms consist of body pains which are often misdiagnosed as psychosomatic. In advanced cases characteristic bone deformities occur and skeletal X-rays show demineralisation of bone.

Osteomalacia is also likely to occur in the elderly. The efficiency of calcium absorption tends to decrease with age, so higher intakes, as much as 900 mg/day, may be necessary for the elderly to remain in calcium balance. Because of ignorance, lack of resources, physical disability with eating and relative immobilisation they are deficient both in calcium and vitamin D. An incidence of 8 per cent has been reported in 200 elderly women consecutively admitted to hospital in Glasgow. Further observations are needed on the frequency of osteomalacia in the elderly in both temperate and warm countries.

Hypercalcaemia

Excess intake of vitamin D can lead to hypercalcaemia, especially in susceptible infants. The widespread tendency to enrich infant foods with vitamin D increases the risk, especially when we know that large inaccuracies do occur in the measurement of milk powder. In the 1950s several cases of infantile hypercalcaemia were diagnosed in Western Europe and North America. This led to a recommendation for considerable reduction in the vitamin D content of infant foods. However, the risk is still present, especially with the availability of highly potent and concentrated forms of vitamin D on the market and the tendency for parents to ask for 'tonics'.

Clinical manifestation of rickets

Bony changes and skeletal deformities are the most striking characteristics of rickets, even though other clinical features like irritability, excessive sweating, refusal to eat and a tendency for bronchopneumonia have been found to be commonly present in the rachitic child. There is extension and widening of the epiphyses, more easily noticed at the lower end of the radius (figure 7.2) and at the costochondral junctions of the ribs. If the disease occurs before the age of 6 months there is also softening of the skull bones. Circumscribed areas in the membranous bones of the skull remain unossified, yielding to pressure with the fingers and giving a characteristic feel, similar to that of pressing on parchment.

During pregnancy marked changes in calcium metabolism occur. The mother has to provide large quantities of calcium for the growing fetus whilst maintaining adequate plasma and bone concentrations of calcium in herself. There is a rise in the plasma concentration of $1\text{-}25\text{-}(OH)_2\text{-}D_3$ as pregnancy advances and this helps to meet the increased need for calcium through enhancing intestinal absorption. In the case of mothers who are deficient in vitamin D, or who have a degree of osteomalacia, the newborn has a tendency for vitamin D deficiency which may progress to hypocalcaemic tetany. Other signs of neonatal and infantile rickets are craniotabes, bossing of the skull, delayed closure of the anterior fontanelle and rickety rosary.

Late signs are bony deformities in lower extremities, like bow-legs or knock-knees, and a transverse depression of the chest which deepens on expiration. All these deformities can be explained by the softening of bones which bend under stress, either that of weight-bearing or by muscle traction. Frontal bossing of the skull, late closure of the anterior fontanelle and various bony deformities are other stigmata of rickets.

Treatment and prevention

Life-threatening situations like hypocalcaemic tetany need to be treated with intravenous calcium 100-200 mg/kg per dose followed by daily oral calcium in the form of calcium chloride 100mg/kg/day divided in three doses. In addition vitamin D 75 µg daily should be administered for 3 weeks followed by 10 µg daily thereafter. Most cases of rickets respond well to oral administration of 125-250 µg of vitamin D daily for a period of 4-6 weeks. Radiological improvement is seen in 2-3 weeks, though biochemical tests continue to remain abnormal for a long time.

As past experience shows, rickets is preventable. The problem is now mainly confined to a section of the community with large families living in slums and inner-city areas. Mothers in such families do not use health or social services and are unresponsive to health visitors. Amongst immigrant families in industrial countries there are added difficulties because of language and cultural differences. Moreover, exposure to sunlight in dull and cold climates and in crowded cities is not always possible. In the mushrooming cities of the developing world the incidence is likely to increase and reach epidemic proportions unless active steps are taken. A multiple approach through education, provision of fortified foods and prophylactic administration of vitamin D is most likely to succeed in such circumstances. Amongst Asian immigrant women prophylactic administration of vitamin D during pregnancy has been shown to improve the calcium status of the infants and to reduce the incidence of neonatal hypocalcaemia.

The discovery of vitamin D as an antirachitic factor was made during a period when several food factors in trace quantities were being identified as essential nutrients for the prevention of specific deficiency diseases. This led to its designation as a vitamin which was reinforced by the demonstration of its presence in natural foods like egg yolk, milk and fish.

Cod liver oil became a convenient form of supplying the vitamin. Later manufacturers of infant foods incorporated the vitamin in their products. It is only recently recognised that solar irradiation is more important in maintaining vitamin D status and is a more effective source of obtaining it. Unlike other fat-soluble vitamins like A, E and K, the liver in man has little ability to store vitamin D. Instead, excess dietary vitamin D may be inactivated metabolically and the products excreted in bile or else converted to 25-(OH)-D_3 which is then secreted back into the blood. On the other hand, cholecalciferol produced in the skin diffuses slowly into the circulation and is bound to vitamin D specific protein in the blood. This slows down its presentation to the liver and so the conversion to 25-(OH)-D_3 is much slower than would be the case if the same amount came from the diet. Molecule for molecule vitamin D formed in the skin is more efficiently utilised than that obtained from the diet.

Development of laboratory methods for the assay of vitamin D metabolites has led to improved understanding of their functions and interactions in several diseases affecting bone growth and calcium metabolism. The role of vitamin D is now conceived in terms of one or more metabolites having endocrine roles in calcium and phosphate homeostasis. For example, bone disease may develop in patients with chronic renal failure, and pharmacologic doses of vitamin D can induce healing of the bone. It is likely that the disturbance of calcium metabolism and the secondary hyperparathyroidism in chronic renal failure are caused by the reduced capacity for producing 1-25-$(OH)_2$-D_3. Similarly, in chronic liver disease rickets and osteomalacia occur which respond to administration of vitamin D. Here defective absorption of vitamin D associated with defective 25-hydroxylation is often the underlying cause.

Two genetically determined types of rickets have been described. One is transmitted as a sex-linked (X-linked) disorder in which the outstanding defect is in the form of renal tubular leak of phosphate, and not any impairment of vitamin D metabolism. Hence the condition does not respond well to vitamin D though partial healing of the bone lesions can occur with high doses. The second, much rarer, disorder is autosomal recessive, and responds well to vitamin D or 1-25-$(OH)_2$-D_3. The genetic defect here is thought to be in the hydroxylation reaction in the kidney. Another genetic variant of the condition is expressed as end organ resistance to 1-25-$(OH)_2$-D_3.

DEFICIENCIES OF VITAMINS OF THE B GROUP

The vitamins of the B group act as co-factors or activators of enzymes and thus have a key role in metabolism. Enzymes involved in metabolic activity vary a great deal in their functions. Some require only their main proteins to be active, others require the presence of co-factors. In some cases these co-factors are simple metallic ions and in others they are more complex molecules. In the latter case they are termed co-enzymes. The vitamins of the B group are mainly co-enzymes or precursors of such co-enzymes.

Most co-enzymes bind loosely to the protein portion of the apoenzyme, but some like thiamine bind more firmly. Some co-enzymes serve as receptors for the products of enzyme reaction. For example, folic acid serves as a receptor of methyl groups and one carbon fragment in the synthesis of purine and in the metabolism of several amino acids. Some co-enzymes act as electron or proton receptors. Thus, riboflavin acts as a receptor of hydrogen atoms in the oxidation-reduction reactions within the mitochondria for the liberation of energy. Some co-enzymes, on the other hand, act as structural supports to the enzyme molecule, exposing the active sites or changing their configuration for optimal chemical reaction without directly participating in reactions.

Deficiencies of vitamins in the B group arise for various reasons. The commonest cause is dietary, caused by either inadequate consumption of food or by eating processed foods in which the vitamin concerned may have been removed or destroyed. It is useful to bear in mind that more than one vitamin can be absent from a deficient diet. Moreover, several B vitamins are used in the metabolism of a common substrate and a deficiency of one will affect the use of another. When food is inadequate, most metabolic processes are slowed, as in clinical malnutrition. The immediate need for specific vitamins may be reduced and vitamin depletion may go unrecognised. On refeeding, signs of deficiency become apparent. Rarer causes of vitamin deficiency are poor intestinal absorption or a deficiency of transport protein needed for the transfer of the vitamin across the gut mucosa. At the cellular level, the co-factors may not be transported across the cell membrane, transport within the cell may be defective, or it may not be converted to the form needed to activate apoenzymes. The co-factor may not bind adequately to the apoenzyme because of a defect in the protein binding site or because some other compound is competing. Deficiencies at the cellular level give rise to abnormal metabolism with the formation of toxic by-products.

The vitamins of the B group are widely distributed in nature. In addition, many of them are synthesised by intestinal bacteria, so that in a healthy individual eating a mixed diet deficiencies are rare. In spite of this, deficiencies reaching epidemic proportions have occurred not very long ago with regard to several vitamins. These are pellagra due to niacin deficiency and beri-beri due to lack of thiamine in the diet. In addition, megaloblastic anaemia of pregnancy caused by deficiency of folic acid is still common in many parts of the developing world today. Both pellagra and beri-beri, which once affected tens of thousands of people, are now on the decline, but the causative factors and the circumstances in which they occur still continue to exist and the potential for future outbreaks remains.

PHYSIOLOGICAL ROLES OF NIACIN (NICOTINAMIDE; NICOTINIC ACID)

Niacin (nicotinamide) is widely distributed in plant and animal foods (Table 7.3). In the liver tryptophan can be converted to niacin and the

Table 7.3 *Sources of niacin (recommended daily intake 6.6 mg/1000 kcal)*

Food	Range (mg/100 g *of edible portion*)
Wheat bran (mainly outer bran)	25.0-46
Wheat flour (70% extraction)	1.0
Wheat flour (British 1956 regulation)	1.5
Rice (lightly milled)	2.0-4.5
Rice (highly milled)	1.0-1.6
Pulses	1.5-3.0
Millets	1.3-3.2
Maize*	0.2-1.5
Sorghum*	2.5-3.5
Ground nuts	16.0
Green leafy vegetables	0.2-1.5

* Staple foods commonly associated with pellagra.

presence of animal protein in the diet helps to protect against deficiency of niacin. Milk, meat and eggs protect against pellagra because of their tryptophan content. However, the conversion process is somewhat inefficient as only about 1.5 per cent of dietary tryptophan is normally converted to niacin. It has been estimated that 60 mg of tryptophan can give rise to 1 mg of niacin. Presumably such a conversion only occurs when tryptophan is in excess and there is a need for niacin. Increasing amounts of tryptophan are first used to achieve nitrogen balance, next to restore blood pyridine nucleotide and then for conversion into niacin. It is customary to take into account both the niacin content of food as well as the amount of tryptophan present in order to determine the 'niacin equivalents' of diets. The amount of niacin required is also related to the total calories consumed and the recommended daily intake is 6.6 niacin equivalents for every 1000 kcal consumed per day. In the normal European diet about half the niacin comes from proteins of animal origin.

In some foods, for example maize and possibly the potato, niacin occurs in a bound form and cannot be absorbed in the gut. It can be liberated from the bound form by treatment with alkali. In Mexico and in the diets of many American Indian communities maize is first treated with lime water prior to use for making tortillas. This helps to liberate niacin from the bound form and increases the amount of utilisable niacin in maize, which explains the low incidence of niacin deficiency in these communities.

Cooking does not destroy niacin except that considerable amounts may be dissolved in the water used for cooking and in the fluids which come out of meats during cooking. If these fluids are discarded instead of being consumed, considerable amounts of niacin may be lost.

Niacin has an essential role in the oxidative mechanisms by which the chemical energy present in the molecules of carbohydrate, fat and protein is liberated and made available for cellular metabolism. It is the precursor of two co-enzymes, NAD (nicotinamide adenine dinucleotide) and NADP (nicotinamide adenine dinucleotide phosphate) which act as hydrogen acceptors in oxidation-reduction reactions. The energy thus released is trapped by the synthesis of high-energy phosphate bonds, and the two co-enzymes also participate in these reactions. Thus, niacin is essential for glycolysis, pyruvate lipid and fat metabolism, and for the synthesis of high energy phosphate compounds.

Pellagra

This is a deficiency disorder caused by lack of niacin. It occurs in poor peasant communities which subsist mainly on maize with very little variety in the diet. The typical clinical features are loss of weight, debility, an erythematous rash characteristically affecting the parts of the body exposed to sunlight, gastrointestinal disturbances and mental changes. Diarrhoea and mental change are not always present, especially in early cases, and often the mental symptoms consist of depression or confusion.

The disease first made its appearance in Europe after the introduction of maize from the New World; together with maize it spread through Europe from Spain to France, Italy, Central Europe, Rumania and Turkey. It later spread into Egypt and tropical Africa. In the first decade of the present century, pellagra was a major disease in the United States, chiefly affecting the poor whites and Negro farm labourers in the South. In 1928, 6969 deaths were recorded from pellagra in the US, and by 1930, 20 000 cases were reported in the state of Georgia alone. Because of its sudden and widespread occurrence it was then thought to be a new epidemic disease of infective origin. Many observers have ascribed the sudden appearance of pellagra in the US to the wide-scale poverty and depression following upon the Civil War, and the development of large milling concerns which marketed finely ground corn flour that looked and tasted better but lacked the germ and its vitamins. The commercial milling of maize in the US made a poor diet even poorer and was the major precipitating factor in the occurrence of pellagra.

Elsewhere similar disasters were recorded. In Rumania, in 1932 55 013 cases were recorded with 1654 deaths. In some villages where maize was the staple food providing something like 75 per cent of total calories, up to 10 per cent of the population suffered from pellagra every Spring. In Lesotho in 1956 it was reported as the most common deficiency disease. During the warm months 15 per cent of the population were affected. In South Africa, in the Bantu reserve areas, about half the patients attending the outpatient clinics have pellagra skin lesions, and more than half of all Bantu patients admitted to mental hospitals are suffering from pellagra in one form or another.

In 1927 the nature of pellagra as a deficiency disorder was established, and the use of milk as a protective food was well known. Liver extract for the treatment of pellagra was available in 1937, and it was not long before niacin was synthesised and widely available. At the same time the governments of many countries instituted preventive programmes. In the US, agricultural extension programmes promoted the development of small farms instead of concentrating on the growing of cotton. In France, government action discouraged the cultivation of maize. In Italy, government subsidies established bakeries to sell bread made from wheat. Similarly, in Egypt maize was gradually replaced by subsidised wheat and farmers were encouraged to mix maize with wheat or millet.

As a result of these measures, pellagra is now on the decline. It is disappearing from the US and countries of southern Europe and the incidence has decreased in the Middle East, even though it continues to remain endemic in small pockets. Africa is now the only continent where pellagra is still a public health problem. It occurs seasonally in a mild form, the dermatitis recurring each year with the growing season. Recurrent and prolonged niacin deficiency in these communities is a cause of chronic diarrhoea and debility. Intercurrent infections in affected individuals are often fatal. After suffering prolonged niacin deficiency and its various complications many ultimately suffer from dementia.

Recently, pellagra has been reported from rural communities in central South India, where maize is not eaten, but sorghum forms the staple diet. Sorghum is high in leucine and the consumption of large amounts of the staple causes an amino-acid imbalance with secondary lack of tryptophan leading to niacin deficiency as a consequence. Sorghum fed as 65 per cent of the diet to dogs has been shown to give rise to black tongue, which is the canine equivalent of human pellagra.

PRESENT TRENDS

Pellagra persists in some vulnerable groups like pregnant women and the elderly in peasant societies subsisting on maize. But the disease is nowhere as widespread as the epidemics which affected the US and southern Europe in the early part of this century. Pellagra is also found in chronic alcoholics and in patients suffering from malabsorption. Tubercular patients who are on poor diets and on long-term treatment with the anti-tubercle drug, isoniazid, may sometimes show clinical signs of deficiency. More recently, pellagrous skin lesions have been reported in the rare Hartnup disease, in which there exists a defect in the transport of tryptophan across mucosal cells resulting in malabsorption and renal loss of this amino acid.

CLINICAL FEATURES OF PELLAGRA

The characteristic features of pellagra, in the skin, the digestive and the nervous system, are commonly superimposed on the general features of undernutrition. Underweight and general debility are often prominent.

The changes in the skin are characteristic and appear symmetrically over those parts of the body which are exposed to the sun. The hands, forearms, face and skin are covered by an erythematous rash resembling sunburn. The lesions burn and itch, and may progress to formation of vesicles which exude fluid causing encrustation and ulceration. Secondary infection often occurs. In long-standing and chronic cases the skin is thick and roughened, with scaling and dark pigmentation (figures 7.4 and 7.5).

Diarrhoea is a common but not constant feature. In affected individuals the small bowel shows varying degrees of villous atrophy. In the advanced case the mouth is sore with a raw tongue and inflamed fissures at the angles of the mouth. The anal canal and rectum may be similarly involved, indicating pathological changes involving the mucous membrane of the lower gastro-intestinal tract and causing the intractable diarrhoea. Anxiety and depression are usually present. In the more severe and acute forms delirium is common and the more chronic and long-standing cases also show signs of dementia. Sensory disturbances are common amongst the latter, with consequent loss of position sense and ataxia.

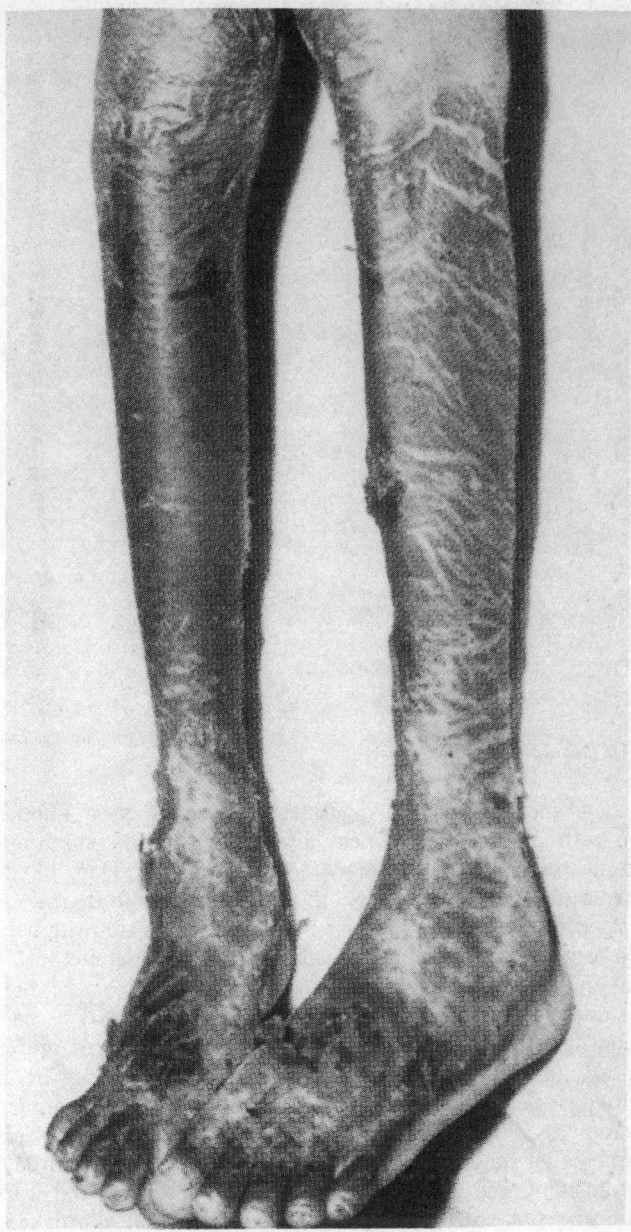

Figure 7.4 Skin rash of pellagra

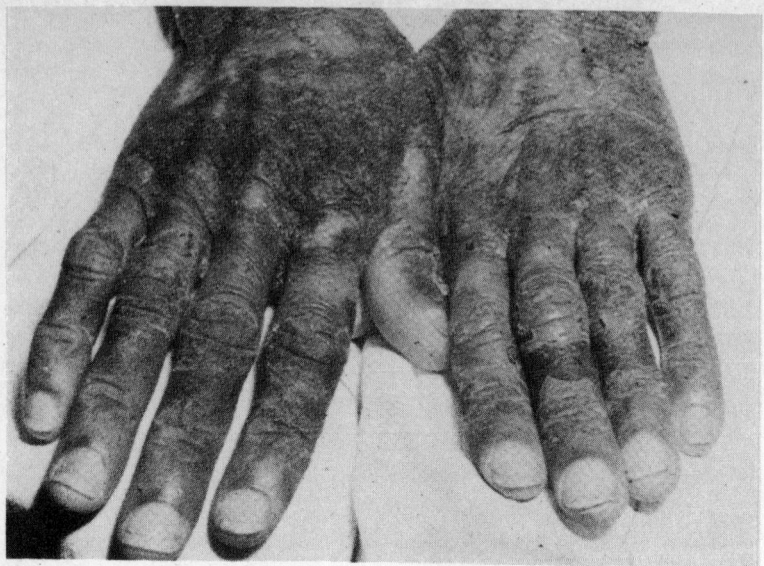

Figure 7.5   Skin rash of pellagra

TREATMENT AND PREVENTION

There is prompt response to nicotinamide 100 mg given 4-hourly by mouth, with general improvement in mental condition and disappearance of diarrhoea and the skin rash. Because of the strong likelihood of other associated deficiencies, other vitamins of the B group and a well-balanced diet are also necessary. In those acute cases with delirium and excitement, both nicotinamide and the other B vitamins need to be given by injection, together with nasogastric feeding.

The disappearance of pellagra from the southern US and many of the countries of Europe demonstrates the effectiveness of preventive measures, and the better understanding of nutritional requirements. In peasant societies, fortification of maize flour with nicotinic acid on a national scale may not be effective because most food is processed in the home. It has been shown that 120 g of ground nuts a day will protect an adult against pellagra. Better extension services and nutrition education in rural societies aimed at the consumption of a mixed diet in addition to national fortification programmes will help to eradicate this eminently preventable deficiency disorder.

Thiamine

All animal and plant tissues contain thiamine, but the more important sources are cereals, peas, beans and other pulses, and yeast. Green vegetables, fruits, dairy products and meat contain appreciable amounts of thiamine, but they are not rich sources (table 7.4).

Table 7.4 *Sources of thiamine (recommended daily intake 0.4 mg/1000 kcal)*

Food	Range (mg/100 g *of edible portion*)
Whole wheat	0.4
Pulses	0.4
Millets	0.4
Rice (home pounded)	0.08-1.4
Rice (parboiled and milled)	0.11
Bran (rice or wheat)	2-4
Milk, cow's	0.04
Eggs	0.10-0.15
Meat	0.16-0.30
Poor sources associated with deficiency	
White bread (70% extraction)	0.05-0.07
Rice (milled)	0.02-0.04

In the cereals, thiamine is chiefly present in the outer layers of the grain which get removed as bran during milling for the making of white flour or rice. Moreover, in the case of rice the removal of outer layers of the grain makes the remaining thiamine more accessible for dissolution in water. Since the common practice is to wash rice prior to cooking, a large part of the remaining thiamine in milled rice is therefore lost during washing. On the other hand, if rice is parboiled, as is the custom in rural communities of South India, the vitamin diffuses into the inner layers of the grain and the losses during milling are minimised.

Thiamine is stable at high temperatures. Losses in cooking occur only when the water used for cooking is discarded, since it contains a large proportion of this highly soluble vitamin. Thiamine is denatured if baking powder is used or if soda is added in the cooking of vegetables. Several foods contain anti-thiamine factors which can alter the biological activity of the vitamin. The viscera of fresh-water fish and shellfish, as well as several micro-organisms, contain substances which catalyse the decomposition of thiamine. These substances are thermolabile and are destroyed during cooking, thereby preserving the vitamin. On the other hand various vegetables and plants also contain anti-thiamine factors which are thermostable and do not get destroyed on cooking.

In many rural Thai communities where thiamine deficiency is endemic studies of nutritional status and food intake have shown that not only is the diet deficient in thiamine, but that the raw fermented fish, which is consumed in large quantities, and the habit of chewing fermented tea leaves as stimulants also make the deficiency worse because of their anti-thiamine activity.

In the healthy individual, thiamine is well absorbed by the intestinal mucosa. At high concentration, absorption is by passive diffusion; at low concentration by active transport. In chronic alcoholics absorption of thiamine is defective, due to associated folate deficiency and malnutrition. Correction of malnutrition and supplementation with folic acid greatly improve thiamine absorption in these individuals.

At the cellular level, thiamine plays an important role in energy metabolism. It participates as a co-enzyme in the metabolism of α-keto acids, like pyruvate and the keto analogues of leucine, isoleucine and valine. It also participates in several important metabolic processes like the pentose phosphate shunt, yielding NADPH. Besides these metabolic roles, thiamine has a specific role in neurophysiology independent of its co-enzyme function.

Beri-beri is a nutritional disorder caused by deficiency of thiamine. The classical descriptions mention two types – wet and dry beri-beri – according to the body systems which are principally involved. The wet type is so called because oedema and symptoms of congestive cardiac failure predominate. In the dry form the prominent signs are those of involvement of the nervous system. The common mode of presentation, however, is the subacute type in which the characteristics of both wet and dry beri-beri are present. A serious form occurs in young breast-fed infants whose mothers are themselves deficient in thiamine. This *infantile form* is at present the commonest variety encountered. It occurs in infants less than 6 months old who are acutely ill with dyspnoea, cold extremities, weak pulse and aphonia. The pseudomeningitic type of beri-beri with strabismus, nystagmus, convulsions and fever has also been described in older infants aged 7–9 months. Depending upon age, abruptness of onset and the severity of the deficiency, various combinations of all the different forms can occur. X-rays show an enlarged heart shadow. There is a dramatic response to injection of thiamine, 10 mg intravenously. Cardiac symptoms resolve in 24–48 hours and neurologic symptoms within 24 hours.

Oedema is also a dominant clinical sign in adult beri-beri. As the disease advances the entire lower extremity and face may become water-logged and swollen. In some cases beri-beri may develop without evident oedema and neurological lesions may predominate. Manifestations may be seen in the motor, sensory as well as the autonomic nervous systems. When beri-beri occurs in association with alcoholism in the adult, the Wernicke-Korsakoff syndrome is the common presenting feature. Again, response to thiamine is dramatic, though motor weakness may take 1-3 months for good recovery.

Beri-beri has been described in various communities in South East Asia where rice is the staple diet. In fact, what maize is to pellagra, rice is to beri-beri, especially the highly milled variety in which thiamine-containing outer layers of the grain have been removed as bran. The disease has also been described in fishing communities on the coast of Newfoundland and Labrador living on a diet principally composed of white wheat flour, salted meat and molasses during the long winter months from October to April.

Early descriptions of beri-beri can be found in medical literature in 1645 and 1835. It was in the last quarter of the nineteenth century that beri-beri suddenly appeared in many countries of South East Asia. It continued as a formidable problem both in extent and severity for about half a century and is now present only in isolated pockets in several South East Asian countries. It would seem that the causative factor in the sudden appearance of beri-beri was the introduction of steam-driven rice mills, so that the use of white, highly milled rice became popular. About the same time several estates and mines employing a large labour force adopted the practice of issuing rice rations as part of the wages for the labourers. Similar practice was also common in the armed forces and barracks. In the affected families, rice was often eaten alone or with little else. For example, it has been noted that rice provided between 2500 and 3000 kcal daily, indicating the large quantities in which it was consumed.

Several observations finally led to the understanding of beri-beri as being a deficiency disease. Epidemiological studies in Malaysia showed that there were three sharply defined communities in the country. The Malays were predominantly agricultural and rural. They grew their own rice and consumed it after home pounding; beri-beri was rare amongst them. The Tamils used parboiled rice, as is the custom in South India. Again beri-beri was rare in this group. The Chinese, on the other hand, were mainly migrant labourers, who consumed white rice provided by their employers. This group was highly prone to beri-beri, with heavy mortality. Further research in the laboratory revealed the protective effect of rice bran. Later thiamine was identified and synthesised. Improved understanding of the nutritional requirements, the wide-scale availability of synthetic thiamine, and fortification of rice by mixing it with the grain coated with thiamine have all helped to reduce the incidence of beri-beri. Socioeconomic development has also resulted in an improved quality of dietary intake and is another factor in the decline of beri-beri.

Riboflavin is widely distributed in nature, dairy produce and foods

Table 7.5 *Sources of riboflavin (recommended daily intake 0.55 mg/1000 kcal)*

Food	Range (mg/100 g of edible portion)
Wheat bran	0.5
Wheat and barley, whole grain	0.12-0.25
Maize, whole grain	0.1
Millets	0.1-0.15
Pulses	0.1-0.3
Fish	0.2-0.4
Meat	0.1-0.3
Eggs	0.3-0.5
Milk - fresh cow's	0.15
Green leafy vegetables	0.05-0.30
Maize meal*	0.02-0.1
Rice - milled*	0.03-0.05
Wheat flour, 70% extraction*	0.03-0.05

* Poor sources.

of animal origin being comparatively richer sources than cereals and plant foods (table 7.5). It is heat-stable and is not destroyed by cooking, apart from the losses which can occur if the water used for cooking is discarded.

Riboflavin is the precursor of the various flavoproteins which act as co-enzymes in many oxidation-reduction reactions, and is essential for tissue respiration. Thus, riboflavin is present in all cells in the form of functioning and active compounds and not as stored nutrient. The liver and kidney contain more than other tissues, but reserves are not great and can be depleted rapidly.

Clinical and biochemical evidence of widespread deficiency is lacking. However, signs of riboflavin deficiency occur in conjunction with other nutritional disorders and should be looked for when other deficiencies occur. Reports from several countries indicate that riboflavin deficiency can be aggravated by the use of oral contraceptives. Similarly, recent reports suggest that phototherapy in jaundiced neonates can induce riboflavin deficiency on account of photodecomposition of riboflavin by blue light. However, administration of the vitamin in pharmacological doses to infants receiving phototherapy is not recommended since *in vitro* studies have shown that riboflavin can alter DNA structure in the presence of light.

Clinically, riboflavin deficiency causes angular stomatitis, broken skin and mucous surfaces around the mouth which may become infected with the fungus *Candida albicans* and develop whitish crusts. The tongue is raw. Eating and swallowing are painful and food intake is further reduced because of it. All the above respond to oral administration of riboflavin 3-10 mg daily.

Pyridoxine

This is widely distributed in nature, with meat, liver, vegetables and the outer coats of cereals being rich sources of the vitamin. It participates as a co-factor in a large number of enzymes concerned with amino acid metabolism, though it is now suggested that the main function of pyridoxine is to stabilise the structure of enzymes rather than act as a co-factor. The metabolic usefulness of pyridoxine can be appreciated by the fact that pyridoxine-carrying enzymes are involved, in one way or another, in the synthesis and catabolism of all amino acids.

A primary deficiency due to inadequate nutrition is rare, but should be suspected in the presence of other nutritional disorders and in malabsorption. Pyridoxine deficiency also occurs in chronic liver disease or uraemia and with the use of drugs which affect the metabolism of the vitamin. In laboratory animals pyridoxine deficiency is characterised by a large number of abnormalities of amino acid metabolism. Poor growth, anaemia, convulsions, decreased antibody formation and renal, hepatic and skin lesions have been described.

Deficiencies can occur through restricted diets, as happened some years ago in infants who were fed a brand of baby food in which pyridoxine had been destroyed through heating. An outbreak of convulsions amongst these infants showed that pyridoxine is an essential nutrient for the developing nervous system. Since then it has been shown that there is a familial tendency in some individuals for higher than normal requirements of pyridoxine. During infancy, they require supplementation with pyridoxine to protect against the risk of seizures which cannot be controlled by the usual anticonvulsants. Some cases of chronic anaemia not responsive to the usual haematinics respond to pyridoxine, indicating that the vitamin overcomes some unknown defect in haemoglobin synthesis. In susceptible women, oral contraceptives are known to induce changes in tryptophan metabolism which are corrected by administration of pyridoxine. Such metabolic disturbances are common in undernourished communities and supplements of pyridoxine may have to be considered in these circumstances. In more recent years it has been shown that many of the neurological side-effects of drugs like isoniazid, cycloserine, hydrallazine and penicillamine can be prevented by pyridoxine. These drugs form complexes with pyridoxine making it unavailable to the tissues.

SUMMARY

This account of vitamin deficiencies serves as a reminder of the dangers of a monotonous diet, especially when the staple has been processed in a way which removes important nutrients. The individual grain of cereal is not only a source of calories, but also contains sufficient vitamins to metabolise the calories present. When this equilibrium is disturbed by technology, as for example removal of the bran, or by bad cooking methods, like discarding the fluids in which the food has been cooked, deficiencies arise. The advent of technology, resulting in the consumption of processed foods, may disturb the balance in nature by selective denaturation of one or more nutrients. There is also the added risk of altering food habits through promotion and through the so-called convenience foods. In the interaction between man and nature for obtaining nutrients, food technology, if not correctly applied, can

Table 7.6 *Vitamin-responsive errors of metabolism*

Vitamin	Disorder	Clinical manifestations	Therapeutic dose (mg)
Thiamine	Leigh's disease (subacute necrotising encephalomyelopathy).	Progressive mental and motor retardation.	100–400
	Wernicke-Korsakoff disease	Alcoholic psychosis.	25–50
	Maple-syrup urine disease variant.	Slow psychomotor development.	5–10
	Thiamine-responsive anaemia.	Megaloblastic anaemia.	20
	Chronic lactic acidosis.	Mental and motor retardation; weakness; ataxia.	5–100
Pyridoxine	Infantile convulsions.	Seizures.	10–50
	Pyridoxine-responsive anaemia.	Hypochromic anaemia.	>10
	Cystathioninuria.	Mental retardation, acromegaly, renal anomalies.	100–500
	Homocystinuria.	Ectopic lens, thrombosis, mental retardation.	25–50
	Xanthurenic aciduria.	Mental retardation.	5–10

give rise to widespread deficiencies as has happened in the past with pellagra and beri-beri, and more recently with infant feeding.

As society changes new trends and eating patterns emerge, partly on account of promotion of new packaged foods and partly due to changes in life-style. In many of the industrialised countries deficiencies of a variety of micronutrients have been recently identified amongst adolescents. These nutritional deficiencies have been attributed to the trend for 'junk' foods which provide flavour and calories without providing the other nutrients in a balanced form, and to the increased consumption of bottled beverages which pander to the taste and provide calories with various additives but lack essential nutrients.

MEGAVITAMIN THERAPY

Several errors in metabolism have been found to respond to pharmacologic doses of vitamins of the B group. A good example is subacute necrotising encephalomyelopathy or Leigh's disease which has features resembling Wernicke's encephalopathy. Children with this progressive disorder have been found to respond to large doses (100-400 mg) of thiamine administered daily. Thiamine plays a similar role in a few other inborn errors of metabolism. Similarly, pyridoxine has been shown to have a therapeutic effect in a variety of metabolic disorders, as set out in table 7.6. The diseases listed in the table have very low priority in the developing world but are mentioned for the sake of completeness.

FURTHER READING

Barker, B. M. and Bender, D. A. (eds) *Vitamins in Medicine*. 4th ed. Heinemann, London, 1980.

Fraser, D. R. Biochemical and clinical aspects of vitamin D function. *Br. Med. Bull.* (1981), **37**, 37-42.

Gopalan, C. and Krishnaswamy, K. Effect of excess leucine on tryptophan niacin pathway and pyridoxine. *Nutr. Rev.* (1976), **34**, 318-19.

Holmes, A. M., Enoch, B. A., Taylor, J. L. and Jones, M. E. Occult rickets and osteomalacia amongst the Asian immigrant population. *Quart. J. Med.* (1973), NS **42**, 1225.

Larsson-Cohn, U. Oral contraceptives and vitamins: a review. *Am. J. Obstet. Gynecol.* (1975), **121**, 84-90.

McLaren, D. S. *Nutritional Ophthalmology*. Academic Press, New York and London, 1980.

Rivlin, R. S. (ed.) *Riboflavin*. Plenum Press, New York, 1975.

Sommer, A. *Nutritional Blindness: Xerophthalmia and Keratomalacia*. Oxford University Press, New York, 1982.

Srikantia, S. G. Human vitamin A deficiency. *World Rev. Nutr. Diet.* (1975), **20**, 184-230.

Tanphaichitr, V. Thiamine. In *Present Knowledge in Nutrition*. The Nutrition Foundation Inc., Washington DC, 1976, pp. 141-7.

Williams, R. R. *Towards the Conquest of Beri-beri*. Harvard University Press, Cambridge, Mass., 1961.

World Health Organization: *Vitamin A Deficiency and Xerophthalmia*. Technical Report Series No. 590. WHO, Geneva, 1976.

Chapter 8

Nutritional Anaemias

Nutritional anaemias comprise the second most common group of deficiency disorders after protein-energy malnutrition. Nutritional anaemia is defined as anaemia which occurs when there is a deficiency of one or more of the essential nutrients required for the synthesis of haemoglobin and the production of erythrocytes. Several nutrients are required for erythropoiesis.

Iron, folic acid, vitamin B_{12}, protein, pyridoxine, vitamin C, copper and possibly vitamin E are all necessary for the proper function of the bone marrow. Iron is an essential component of haemoglobin and a large proportion of nutritional anaemia in the world is caused by its deficiency. Iron deficiency tends to be most common when the intake is not enough to meet the demands of growth, e.g. in pregnancy, during infancy and at adolescence. Infections and parasitic infestations are also important; they may interfere with the activity of the marrow, or increase erythropoiesis by causing blood loss or haemolysis. Iron deficiency also occurs in malabsorption syndromes.

Anaemia due to deficiency of folic acid and vitamin B_{12} is much less common. Both folic acid and B_{12} play a key role in cellular metabolism and are needed for the normal development of the erythrocytes in the bone marrow. Folic acid deficiency is more common than that of vitamin B_{12}, and is mostly seen during pregnancy, when the demands of the fetus are added to those of the mother. Apart from pregnancy, deficiencies of folic acid and B_{12} are rare except in malabsorption and in certain diseases of the bowel as, for example, tropical sprue.

PREVALENCE

Anaemia is a common cause of hospital admissions in infants and young children in most of the developing world. In some countries of tropical Africa up to 4 per cent of paediatric admissions are for anaemia, a figure equivalent to that for admissions due to protein-energy malnutrition; the mortality from anaemia can be as high as 9-10 per cent. The frequency of anaemia in out-patients is even higher. Of 5000 patients attending the teaching hospital in Dar-es-Salaam, the mean haemoglobin value amongst 2539 men was 8.85 g/100 ml. Among 2108 women it was 7.86 g/100 ml, and in 853 children in the age group 1-5 years it was 6.78 g/100 ml. In Mauritius, anaemia is the second most important cause of admissions to hospital and in Sierra Leone up to 40 per cent of adult females suffer from it.

Community studies have been few and scattered. In one detailed study spread over seven countries of South America it was found that iron deficiency occurred in 48 per cent of pregnant women as compared with 21 per cent non-pregnant women, and in 3 per cent of the males of the same age groups. Anaemia, defined as haemoglobin less than 11 g/100 ml, was found in 38.5 per cent of pregnant women, 17.3 per cent of non-pregnant women and 3.9 per cent of men. The prevalence of folic acid and vitamin B_{12} deficiency was much lower and these deficiencies seemed to occur only during pregnancy.

In the Gambia, in one longitudinal study, 473 rural children under the age of 5 years were examined at intervals of 3 months for a period of 26 months. In that community the common practice is to breast feed all children exclusively for 4-6 months, after which cereal pap is introduced and gradually supplemented with sauces of fish, ground nuts or green leaves and boiled rice. The mean haemoglobin value under the age of 1 month was found to be 15.4 g/100 ml. It fell as the children grew older, reaching 9.0 g/100 ml at the age of 15-24 months, after which there was a slow improvement. These values are lower than those of London children in the worst years of the depression in the 1930s and of poor Aberdeen children quoted below. A well-marked seasonal cycle was observed in the Gambia. There was a sharp decline in haemoglobin values in the latter part of the wet season, indicating that malaria is a key aetiological factor in this age group. In another study of anaemia in rural women in the Gambia a high frequency of iron deficiency was observed. In this group there was a strong association between anaemia and three independent variables-pregnancy, heavy menstrual periods and splenomegaly.

A cross-sectional study of haemoglobin values in 726 children under the age of 5 years in several coastal villages in Tanzania showed that anaemia was as common as in the Gambia. The mean haemoglobin was 8.3 g/100 ml in the first 6 months of life, increasing slowly to reach a mean of 9.2 g/100 ml between the ages of 5 and 6 years. Again malaria appeared to be implicated. For example, in the city of Dar-es-Salaam, where malaria transmission is considerably less, the mean haemoglobin values were higher - 10 g/100 ml in the age group 5-6 years.

Forty infants under the age of 6 months with severe anaemia were studied in Dar-es-Salaam. Apart from six who suffered from sickle cell anaemia, all had iron deficiency with little or no iron stores in the bone marrow. A large majority were born to mothers who had received no antenatal care during pregnancy. It was thought that many of these infants were born with poor iron stores and could not cope with the requirements of growth. Episodes of malaria made the existing deficiency worse and precipitated acute anaemia.

Collaborative studies under the auspices of the World Health Organisation indicate that nutritional anaemia affects between 10 and 20 per cent of the populations of the developing countries. The most common cause is iron deficiency, but often deficiencies of folic acid and B_{12} are also simultaneously present, especially in pregnant women (table 8.1).

Table 8.1 *Prevalence of nutritional anaemia in the developing world*

Africa
    6-17% adult males.
    15-50% adult females.
    30-60% children under the age of 15 years.

Asia
    10% adult males.
    30-50% adult females. The rates are higher amongst pregnant women reaching 80-90% in certain regions of India, Pakistan and Bangladesh.
    50% children. The rates are higher in children under the age of 2 years.

Central and South America
    5-15% adult males.
    10-35% adult females. The rates are higher, up to 50%, amongst pregnant women.
    15-50% infants.

Such cross-sectional data are becoming available for many communities, indicating the extensive prevalence of anaemia. Even though there are no symptoms from the anaemia it does contribute to ill-health and reduces productivity. In malarious areas, control measures result in better average levels of haemoglobin. This was the experience in Tanzania after instituting control measures. Also community surveys in India, where malaria eradication programmes have been in operation since the 1960s, show higher haemoglobin levels compared to communities where malaria is holo-endemic. A cross-sectional study in 544 rural Punjabi children showed a mean haemoglobin level of 11.0 g/100 ml under the age of 6 months, falling to 9.2 g/100 ml at age 18-24 months and rising again to 10.5 g/100 ml at 3 years.

In many affluent societies of Western Europe nutritional anaemia used to be a major public health problem until quite recently. In 1935 a survey of 3500 individuals from the poorer classes in Aberdeen showed that between the ages of 5 and 23 months the frequency of anaemia was 41 per cent and in 7 per cent the haemoglobin level was less than 10.2 g/100 ml. Between the ages of 2 and 5 years, 32 per cent had haemoglobin levels below 11 g/100 ml. After this age slow improvement occurred until adolescence when, amongst 246 pubertal girls, 1 per cent had haemoglobin levels below 9.6 g/100 ml. Anaemia was not a problem among adult men; women tended to have lower haemoglobin values, especially during pregnancy when 17.5 per cent showed values of less than 9.6 g/100 ml. Thus, three age groups were identified as being at risk; *viz.* infancy, adolescence especially in girls, and pregnancy. Since then there has been a marked improvement. Recently a mean haemoglobin value of 11.0 g/100 ml has been recorded in Bristol children between the ages of 3 and 24 months and in Cardiff children a mean value of 12.0 g/100 ml in the second year rising to 12.4 g/100 ml at 5 years has been reported.

The general improvements in diet and in health standards have largely contributed to the falling incidence of anaemia in British children. A similar improvement has also been found in pregnant women since 1940, though early prophylaxis with iron and folic acid has also been responsible for the fall in the incidence of anaemia of pregnancy.

AETIOLOGICAL FACTORS

Iron deficiency

Iron plays an important role in the physiology of the body because of its unique ability to give up or accept electrons and oxygen. This enables a rapid change from the ferrous (reduced) to the ferric state (oxidised form) with no expenditure of energy. It has thus a central role in respiration both in the take-up of oxygen in the lungs and its utilisation at the cellular level.

A large number of foods contain iron (table 8.2). The concentration varies in accordance with soil conditions so that a range occurs in most vegetable foods. All food iron is present in two main forms:

(1) Inorganic or non-haem iron, which occurs as ferric hydroxide complexes loosely bound with proteins, amino acids or organic acids. Prior to absorption, this form of iron must be split from its combination with organic molecules and reduced to the ferrous state. It must be then converted to soluble complexes (chelates) by

Table 8.2 *Iron content of common foods (recommended intake 10 mg/day)*

Food	Range (mg/100 g)
Liver, raw	6.0-14.0
Beef, mutton, raw	2.0- 4.3
Fish (raw)	0.5- 1.0
Eggs (whole, fresh)	2.0- 3.0
Pulses	1.9-14.0
Millets (raw)	4.0- 5.4
Cereals	9.0 mg
Wheat flour (high extraction)	3.0- 7.0
Wheat flour (low extraction)	0.7- 1.5
Green vegetables	0.4-18.0
Potatoes and root vegetables	0.3- 2.0
Milk	0.1- 0.4
Soya flour	12.0 mg

combining with amino acids, polypeptides or sugars. This happens during acid-pepsin digestion in the stomach. Reducing substances like vitamin C help in absorption. On the other hand, presence of phytates can result in the formation of insoluble salts and prevent absorption. For this reason cereals are a poor source, in spite of their rich iron content. Egg yolk also suffers from a similar disadvantage because of its phosphate content.

(2) Haem iron, which is bound to porphyrin in haemoglobin and myoglobin. Its absorption is not affected by phytate or phosphate or ascorbic acid. Haem iron is absorbed intact into the intestinal epithelial cells and the iron is split off from the haem moiety within the epithelial cell.

Several ingenious studies with radioactive iron biologically incorporated into foods have helped our understanding of the absorptive mechanisms and of the availability of iron from various foods. Thus, iron is better absorbed from veal and fish as compared to wheat. The least absorption is from beans, spinach and maize. In general, iron absorption from meals based predominantly on plant foods is quite low (1-5 per cent) and absorption from diets containing adequate amounts of animal protein is higher (8-10 per cent). A diet providing 10-12 mg of iron per day, and in which at least 40 per cent of the iron comes from meat, will provide adequate amounts for normal adults. The average diet in the UK in 1976 provided 12 mg of iron daily. Of this 15 per cent was obtained from white bread and another 23 per cent came from pastries and cereal products. Meat provided about a quarter of the total iron intake, so that more than half the iron intake came from bread, wheat flour and meat. In the average diet haem iron contributes only 1-3 mg of iron per day and in the poorer peasant communities even less. Non-haem iron which forms the bulk of the dietary iron is far less available.

Factors influencing absorption of iron are largely those contained in foodstuffs. Inhibitors as well as promoters of iron absorption are present in most foods. Inhibitors like phytates, phosphates and tannins are more common in foods of vegetable origin. The role of tannin has been described only recently. It has been shown that tannin in tea forms insoluble tannate complexes with non-haem iron which cannot be absorbed. The seed coats of legumes, condiments and spices contain appreciable amounts of tannin. On the other hand, ascorbic acid and animal protein, especially meat, help the absorption of iron.

A large proportion of iron is absorbed in the duodenum and the efficiency of absorption decreases from the proximal to the distal parts of the duodenum. Absorption can also occur in the jejunum and proximal ileum. Colonic absorption of soluble ferrous iron has been demonstrated but it is doubtful whether the colon is a significant site of absorption. All ferric iron in the food must be converted to the soluble ferrous form before it can be absorbed. This process commences in the stomach and continues in the small intestine. In people with achlorhydria and in patients after gastrectomy, iron absorption is decreased. For example, achlorhydria decreases iron absorption by up to 50 per cent. Such individuals cannot increase absorption when iron deficient, and must be given parenteral iron.

Iron taken up by the brush border of the enterocyte rapidly passes into the cell. The quantity of iron transferred from the lumen into the enterocytes depends upon the availability of receptors on the brush border. The receptors compete for iron with the ligand in the gut lumen. Some ligands bind to iron and keep it in solution, thereby promoting its absorption, and others inhibit absorption by precipitating iron. Unlike inorganic iron, haem is not bound to ligands. It can enter the enterocyte directly where the haem molecule is broken down and iron released (figure 8.1).

Within the enterocyte iron is bound to specific carriers and transferred to the serosal side. Here it is delivered to plasma transferrin. Excess iron in the cell which is not transferred to plasma transferrin is taken up by apoferritin and stored as ferritin. Ferritin iron constitutes a slowly exchangeable pool with a half-life of about 4 days. It can be mobilised by combining with carriers. On the other hand it can be lost by the desquamation of cells. Formerly it was believed that iron absorption was determined by the amount of ferritin deposited in the mucosal cell. This 'mucosal block' theory is now being discarded. The presently

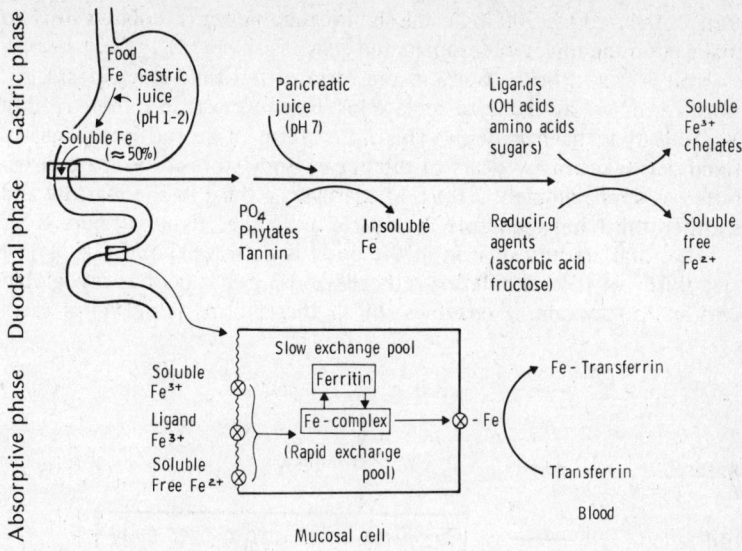

Figure 8.1 The physiology of iron absorption

accepted view is that ferritin deals with excess intracellular iron not transferred to plasma.

The gut mucosa plays a regulatory role in iron absorption which depends upon the saturation of the mucosal cells with iron. Several homeostatic mechanisms have been identified as influencing iron absorption. Thus, the state of repletion of body stores, degree of erythropoiesis and hypoxia influence iron absorption but the exact mechanisms regulating absorption are not yet fully understood.

In adults with iron deficiency, 20 per cent of labelled iron can be absorbed compared to less than 10 per cent in controls. In the average Western diet providing between 10 and 15 mg of iron per day, only 5-10 per cent is absorbed. Absorption decreases with advancing age, especially after 60, when iron deficiency is common.

Iron absorbed into the blood stream is carried by transferrin which is a specific plasma protein of the β-globulin group. In the adult male, 20 mg of iron is liberated daily from catabolised erythrocytes and is recycled by the transport system to the bone marrow for incorporation into new red blood cells. The daily turnover of plasma iron is about 35 mg; only a small portion of it is derived from the diet even when absorption has been at a maximum. The total amount of functioning tissue iron in the adult is 300 mg and a significant amount is replaced daily to make good the losses in desquamated cells.

Iron is stored in the body in the form of ferritin and haemosiderin. Both forms are available to replace lost iron but ferritin is more readily available than haemosiderin. This latter form of stored iron is nearly fixed and takes many years to disappear. Body stores of iron are distributed as approximately a third in the liver, a third in the marrow and another third between spleen, muscle and other tissues (figure 8.2).

The total amount of iron in the body is between 3 and 5 g, almost two-thirds of it in circulating red cells and 3-5 per cent as myoglobin and in iron-containing enzymes. In all these forms it occurs as haem

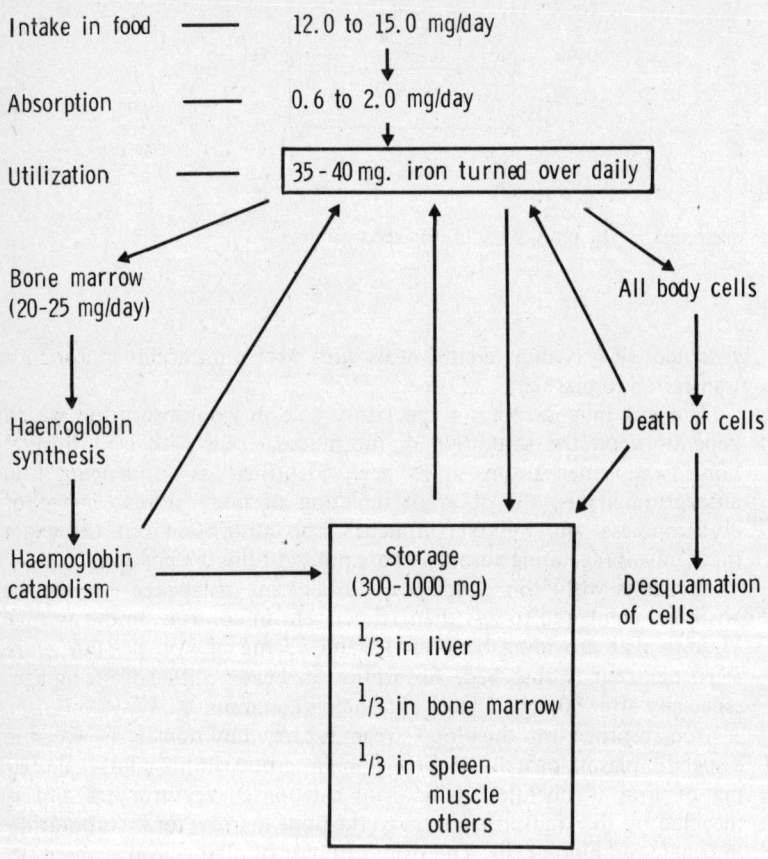

Figure 8.2 Body stores and turnover of iron

iron. The remaining 30 per cent is present as non-haem iron, bound to protein for the purpose of storage and transport.

During pregnancy the placenta is a site of significant iron transfer, especially in the later stages. No significant amount of transferrin crosses the placenta so presumably iron is removed from transferrin and taken up by placental receptors, from whence it is then transferred to the fetus. The iron requirements of pregnancy are approximately 2.4 mg/day over the whole 9 months and the total cost of pregnancy is about 1000 mg (table 8.3). Because of the requirements of pregnancy and

Table 8.3 *Iron requirements in pregnancy (mg)*

Basal losses	220
Increase in maternal red cell mass	500
Requirements of the fetus	290
In the placenta	25
Total requirements for the whole pregnancy	1,035

losses in menstrual blood, the iron requirements of a woman in the reproductive period of life are at least twice those of a man or of a post-menopausal woman.

At birth, the normal full-sized infant has a high concentration of iron in the liver, almost 10 times that at 1-3 years of age. The total iron content of such an infant is 250 mg (75 mg/kg) of which 150 mg is present in the red cell mass, 50 mg in tissues and 50 mg as storage iron. A large proportion of iron endowment at birth is in the form of haemoglobin iron. During the first 4 months of life the decreasing haemoglobin mass makes iron available for the needs of the growing tissues. If iron stores at birth are normal, iron absorption has to be enough to provide only for the basal losses. There is growing evidence that the iron content of breast milk is adequate for the purpose and that breast feeding has a protective effect against iron deficiency. Delayed clamping of the cord after birth can increase the blood volume of the newborn by as much as 100 ml, most of which would be broken down and augment the body stores of iron. In communities where iron deficiency is common, maternal anaemia and poor body stores can lead to a low haemoglobin concentration in the cord blood, poor fetal stores of iron and even anaemia in early infancy. For example, at the maternity hospital in Dar-es-Salaam, 100 consecutive cord blood samples showed a mean haemoglobin value of 9.5 g/100 ml (range 6.2-13.8 g/100 ml). The mean haemoglobin of the mothers was 6.8 g/100 ml. Clearly, many of these infants cannot be expected to have normal tissue stores of iron and are likely to suffer from anaemia in infancy.

In the first 2 years of life there is rapid growth, so that birth weight doubles by the age of 6 months, trebles by the age of 1 year and quadruples by the age of 2 years. There is a parallel increase in blood volume and muscle mass and the demand for iron is high in this age group. The requirement during the first year of life is for 200 mg decreasing to 100 mg by the third year. It continues at that level until the ninth year when the requirement increases concomitant with the growth spurt of puberty. Thus, the body needs of iron are high at two periods of life, infancy and pregnancy. In both, the requirements are several times those of the adult male.

Folic acid and vitamin B_{12}

Both these vitamins are necessary in purine metabolism and for the synthesis of DNA. Deficiency causes a characteristic change in nuclear morphology, and the tissues with the highest rate of cell multiplication are affected first. Deficiency is accentuated by any condition causing increased rate of cell multiplication. Thus it is commonly associated with pregnancy, infancy, lactation and adolescence. For the same reason, haemolysis and certain parasitic infections make marginal deficiency more acute by increasing the requirements.

The commonest form in which deficiency presents itself is megaloblastic anaemia. Severe megaloblastic anaemia is infrequent in affluent societies and occurs usually as a complication of a co-existing main disease. No accurate figures are available of the prevalence of megaloblastic anaemia in the tropics, and it is possible that the frequency and importance of megaloblastic anaemia have been under-estimated. Deficiency can go undiagnosed because it occurs without anaemia or is masked by another haematological or medical disorder.

Megaloblastic anaemia due to deficiency of folic acid is most common in pregnancy. In developed countries the incidence of megaloblastic anaemia in pregnant women attending antenatal clinics is between 2.5 and 5 per cent. The incidence of megaloblastic change in the bone marrow and of low serum folate levels is 8-10 times higher. The information is very scanty with regard to developing countries and present evidence suggests that the incidence of megaloblastic anaemia in pregnancy may be between 20 and 50 per cent.

In children megaloblastic anaemia is rare in well-nourished communities, except as part of the malabsorption syndrome. In developing countries, megaloblastic anaemia is known to occur in protein-energy malnutrition, especially in pastoral communities living on goat's milk, which is low in folic acid. With cow's milk, boiling or pasteurisation can result in the loss of 75 per cent of the folate.

Folate deficiency is a commoner cause of megaloblastic anaemia than deficiency of B_{12}, because body stores of folate are more easily depleted than those of B_{12} and even a minor degree of dietary lack or malabsorption can precipitate deficiency. Alcohol and several drugs, including anti-malarials, can interfere with folic acid metabolism and cause a deficiency.

In most foods, folic acid (pteroylglutamic acid) occurs in the form of polyglutamates. But only pteroylmonoglutamic acid can be utilised, hence hydrolysis of the polyglutamates of the food is necessary. This occurs in the mucosal cells of the small intestine. Many of the naturally occurring folates are labile and easily destroyed by prolonged cooking. In the average British diet 16-24 per cent of free folate is derived from cow's milk. Liver is a rich source so that even one meal of liver can make a significant contribution to the week's intake. The relative availability of the polyglutamate forms of folic acid and pteroylmonoglutamic acid is not yet clear. On present evidence it would appear that the polyglutamate forms are not as available to the body as pteroylmonoglutamic acid. Approximately half the folate present in food is retained and the remainder excreted regardless of whether it is ingested as mono- or polyglutamate.

Amongst the poorer communities of the developing world, fresh vegetables are the main source of folic acid. However, the increasing cost of fresh vegetables coupled with their relative scarcity in certain seasons may limit intake of the vitamin. Lentils are another good source but they require prolonged cooking. Unless soaked overnight, and preferably sprouted prior to cooking, the prolonged cooking is likely to destroy the folic acid.

Vitamin B_{12} exists in nature only as a product of synthesis by microorganisms. Fruit, vegetables, cereals and cereal products are devoid of B_{12} and the usual dietary sources are meat and meat products and, to a lesser extent, milk. Because of its predominantly animal source, strict vegetarians invariably develop B_{12} deficiency over a period of many years, unless they take special measures to avoid it.

In some species such as, for example, the ruminants, vitamin B_{12} is exclusively synthesised by the bacteria in the gut. In the human this source is inadequate to meet the requirements of the body, and the vitamin must be supplied in the food. Vitamin B_{12} occurs in nature as linked to protein by means of peptide bonds, and is liberated during cooking and digestion.

For absorption vitamin B_{12} must first combine with the intrinsic factor secreted by the cells of the gastric mucosa. The vitamin B_{12} –

intrinsic factor complex then attaches itself to receptor sites on the mucosal cells of the ileum where vitamin B_{12} is absorbed.

The average diet in the UK provides approximately 5 µg/day of vitamin B_{12}. Little is known about average intakes in developing countries and one estimate puts it as between 0.5 and 2.0 µg. The maximum amount of the vitamin that can be absorbed at any given meal is between 1.5 and 3.5. µg. The intake from three well-balanced meals in one day will thus provide enough vitamin B_{12} to meet the daily requirement of 2-5 µg. Even the grossly inadequate diet consumed by some old people contains enough vitamin B_{12} to prevent anaemia and therefore a nutritional cause for a deficiency is rare.

Studies of erythropoiesis in megaloblastic anaemia indicate that in this state ineffective erythropoiesis may represent as much as 63 per cent of total erythroid activity. The bone marrow is capable of sustaining erythropoiesis at up to seven times the normal rate, but the proliferative effort only results in an increased number of abnormal cells, which may be destroyed within the marrow or, if delivered into the circulation, are short-lived. The net result is that cell destruction is far greater than erythropoiesis, with consequent anaemia.

Pregnancy and lactation increase the requirements of both folate and vitamin B_{12} in the same way as they do for iron. Hence megaloblastic anaemia more commonly occurs in pregnancy, especially in communities where marginal deficiencies occur. In one study of 1000 pregnant women in South India almost a third had a haemoglobin concentration of less than 10 g/100 ml. Evidence of macrocytosis in the blood smear was found in 27 per cent, but the bone marrow showed a megaloblastic picture in 60 per cent. The mean concentration of serum folate was significantly lower than in female controls. Many of the pregnant subjects showed clinical signs of nutritional deficiency like glossitis (19 per cent), stomatitis (7 per cent) and koilonychia (8 per cent). Serum folate levels were particularly low in such cases, indicating that several deficiencies co-existed. It is important that body stores of nutrients are made up after a pregnancy because if the diet is inadequate and a deficiency continues until the next pregnancy, the baby will be born with poor body stores. As we have seen, such a continuing deficiency occurs with regard to iron, resulting in low haemoglobin values of cord blood, poor fetal stores of iron, and anaemia in infancy. Recovery of body stores of iron, folic acid and other nutrients may occur during school age, but body requirements increase again to sustain the growth spurt at adolescence. In many peasant communities early marriage and child-bearing is the rule, so that if a deficiency persists at adolescence it is transmitted to the offspring. Thus, in poor communities nutritional anaemia, especially anaemia due to iron deficiency, tends to be carried forward from one generation to another.

Folic acid deficiency also occurs in pre-term infants. Demands of growth exceed intake of the vitamin and they use up their tissue stores which, in any case, may be less than normal.

At birth serum and red cell folate levels are high in both pre- and full-term infants compared with adult values. In the cord blood the concentration of folic acid is about three times that in the maternal blood, indicating active transfer of folic acid from the maternal to the fetal side of the placenta. Similarly there is preferential transfer of vitamin B_{12} to the fetus. It is estimated that 0.2 µg/day of vitamin B_{12} is transferred from the mother to the fetus during the latter half of pregnancy. Folate levels drop rapidly soon after birth in all infants, but the drop in value is more rapid and more severe in pre-term infants. The newborn infant's requirement for folate in milk feeds is 20–50 µg/1, and most proprietary milk formulae also provide the same amount. Warming the feeds after reconstitution for the purpose of sterilising will destroy the folate. For example, it has been shown that boiling for as little as 5 seconds reduces the folate content by 50 per cent. Folate deficiency should be suspected in all anaemic pre-term babies and particularly in those with very low birth weights or those with a history of feeding difficulties.

In infants, repeated infections are known to cause anaemia with megaloblastic changes in the bone marrow. Similarly haemolysis due to any cause, e.g. malaria or sickle cell anaemia, increases the requirements of folic acid to meet the needs of a hyperactive marrow.

Megaloblastic anaemia due to deficiency of vitamin B_{12} is comparatively rare and is usually restricted to undernourished communities who are on a predominantly vegan diet, for religious or cultural reasons. A megaloblastic anaemia caused by the fish tapeworm *Diphyllobothrium latum* is found in Scandinavia, Japan and the Great Lakes region of the United States and Canada and is due to a deficiency in the host caused by the tapeworm which diverts the vitamin in the gut lumen for its own use. In heavily infested areas of Finland up to 27 per cent of the population are known to be carriers, and one in 50 such carriers is known to develop megaloblastic anaemia.

Loss of nutrients

There are no physiological mechanisms for the excretion of iron except through the desquamation of cells lining the gut and of the skin. Hence the amount of iron in the body is mainly controlled by absorption.

The main cause of loss of iron from the body is through chronic blood loss – either from heavy menstrual periods or from the gut. In the tropics hookworm and *Trichuris* infestations are well-known causes of iron deficiency anaemia. The adult worm is firmly attached to the mucosa of the gut and obtains blood from the host for its own needs of oxygen and glucose. Experiments with labelled iron in volunteers indicates that in heavy infections considerable quantities of blood may be lost (table 8.4). In such cases the losses cannot be recovered from the daily diet and over a period of time a debilitating chronic anaemia develops. As a general rule, above a critical load of 2000 eggs of hookworm per g of faeces severe iron deficiency and anaemia are likely to occur.

Table 8.4 *Faecal blood losses due to intestinal parasites (ml/day)*

	Per parasite	Per 100 eggs in 1 g faeces
Necator americanus	0.02–0.07	2.1
A. duodenale	0.14–0.26	4.4
Trichuris	0.005	0.25

Several cultural practices in traditional societies can contribute to iron deficiency through bleeding at periods when the body needs of iron are greatest. In several traditional societies of tropical Africa the cutting of the uvula as a treatment for cough or for its prophylaxis is a common practice. In many instances the procedure is carried out when the infant is 3 days old and in some communities up to 96.2 per cent of infants have undergone the procedure before the age of 6 months. Similarly female circumcision is widely practised in tropical Africa. Blood loss at the time of the operation, and the recurrent oozing of blood from the site, may contribute to iron deficiency, especially if body stores are poor or during periods of rapid growth.

Where malaria is endemic it is a major cause of anaemia. Haemolytic anaemia is a common complication of pregnancy in Nigeria and responds to treatment with anti-malarial drugs and folic acid. It has been postulated that haemolysis in malaria is always in excess of the destruction of erythrocytes by the malarial parasites. This is because of an immunological response to malaria by the host. The body stores of iron, folic acid and other nutrients soon get exhausted because of an overactive marrow and because the poor diet supplies very little.

In addition to the direct effect on the erythrocytes, repeated malarial infection is also responsible for a chronic anaemia associated with enlarged spleen. In the so-called tropical splenomegaly syndrome, parasitaemia is scanty or absent and the red cell morphology resembles that of iron deficiency. Studies with labelled iron have shown a high plasma turnover of iron. A large number of erythrocytes are trapped in the enlarged spleen and represent a considerable portion of the red cell mass, which may be between 50 and 75 per cent of the total pool. It is likely that sequestration of such a large number of erythrocytes results in active erythropoiesis by the marrow, using up the available stores of iron and folic acid.

Folic acid deficiency at times associated with a deficiency of vitamin B_{12} is common in tropical sprue. Here morphological changes in the mucosa due to the enteropathy combine with excessive bacterial growth in the bowel to precipitate deficiency in the host. Response to treatment with folic acid and vitamin B_{12} is rapid. Those patients who do not respond to treatment with the vitamins alone may require the addition of antibiotics.

In conclusion, nutritional anaemias are the second largest group of nutritional disorders after protein-energy malnutrition. The individual is most vulnerable at those periods of life when the requirements for nutrients are increased because of the demands of growth. In many parts of the tropics nutritional anaemia is particularly common on account of inadequate nutrition and super-added parasitic or helminthic infections which further increase the requirements of nutrients. In many of the affluent societies of Western Europe, nutritional anaemia used to be a public health problem not so very long ago. The present improvement has been brought about by better standards of health care, especially during infancy and pregnancy, and better nutrition, together with public health measures.

FURTHER READING

Baker, S. J. and De Maeyer, E. M. Nutritional anaemia: its understanding and control with special reference to the work of the World Health Organisation. *Am. J. Clin. Nutr.* (1979), **32**, 368-417.

World Health Organisation. *The prevalence of nutritional anaemia in women in developing countries.* Document FHE/79.3. World Health Organisation, Geneva, 1979.

Yusufji, D., Mathan, V. and Baker, S. J. Iron, folate and vitamin B_{12} nutrition in pregnancy: a study of 1000 women from South India. *Bull. Wld. Hlth. Org.* (1973), **48**, 15-22.

Chapter 9

Community Programmes for Better Nutrition

In spite of major scientific advances in the subject of nutrition, the overall burden of malnutrition in the world has not changed much, and may have even become worse during the last decade. It has been often stressed that if only the available knowledge were to be uniformly applied, there would be very little malnutrition left. Thus the main constraint will appear to be our inability in creating viable national systems for delivering nutritional information and care to the majority of people, especially in the developing countries. Several years ago the world community became aware of the fact that in China, with a population equal to one-fifth of the total world population, there was very little malnutrition. This large nation, once described as 'the sick man of Asia', and with only 20 per cent of its land surface arable, had at last succeeded in feeding her people. Since then several reports on China show that progress has been achieved in many directions. Agricultural productivity has improved, though still continuing to be labour-intensive; the general standard of health has improved remarkably and there is an efficient system of distribution with local self-sufficiency. Are these experiences and achievements applicable to the rest of the developing world with different politico-social systems, diverse cultural and historical experiences and operating from differing planes of technological development?

About the same time small-scale projects of health and integrated development came to be established in several countries. These projects have provided valuable records and experiences of setting up systems of care for hitherto unreached populations. Recently a study of ten such projects in different parts of the world has shown that a marked improvement in health and nutrition has occurred amongst the beneficiaries. In these experiences lies the hope of modifying existing systems of delivery of care in ways that would ensure improvement in the general nutritional status of the community. This chapter is addressed to the district health team in the average developing country who are likely to be confronted by many of the clinical problems described in the preceding chapters.

THE NEED FOR A DISTRICT INVENTORY OF NUTRITION INTERVENTIONS

In almost all countries there exist a variety of national programmes and strategies for the improvement of the general nutritional status of the population. These vary from food distribution schemes and feeding programmes (school meals, mid-day meals, on-the-spot or take-home feeding programmes) to the issuing of food supplements to vulnerable groups like pregnant and lactating women and children, ration cards, food subsidies and fair-price shops. More recently several countries have set up programmes for the preservation of breast feeding. It is necessary to prepare an inventory of all current nutrition programmes in the district, including an assessment of their effectiveness in reaching out to those in need. The purpose of such an inventory is to determine for each of the programmes the resources currently used, the intended beneficiaries, the geographic outreach, the key personnel and their training needs as well as the political and administrative support.

In a given district the nutrition activities and programmes are part of the nutrition system which is the channel through which nutrients pass from suppliers (local production and imports), through distributors and the processing media to the consumer. The effectiveness of this system in reaching families and communities at the periphery will determine the state of nutrition of the population in general and of the economically weaker sections in particular. In most developing countries the indigenous components of the nutrition system are insignificant. There are low yields in agricultural production, there is wastage in storage, there is inequity in distribution and there are problems of transportation. On the other hand, unemployment, lack of land resources and of technical know-how reduce the ability of large segments of the population to provide their nutritional requirements. Nutrition projects, often funded by international aid agencies but now increasingly through national resources, are intended to help strengthen and buttress the nutrition system so as to improve the supply of nutrients for the target groups.

In most countries the national health system provides the major outlets for a variety of nutritional intervention programmes. Thus, there are services for providing curative care for the severely malnourished, and health surveillance clinics like the antenatal and under-5s clinics where preventive measures can be applied for the promotion of adequate growth and nutrition as well as for protecting the undernourished from severe malnutrition. These services also provide the main framework for the promotion of breast feeding in the community. Thus the health centre and the satellite sub-centres are useful springboards for monitor-

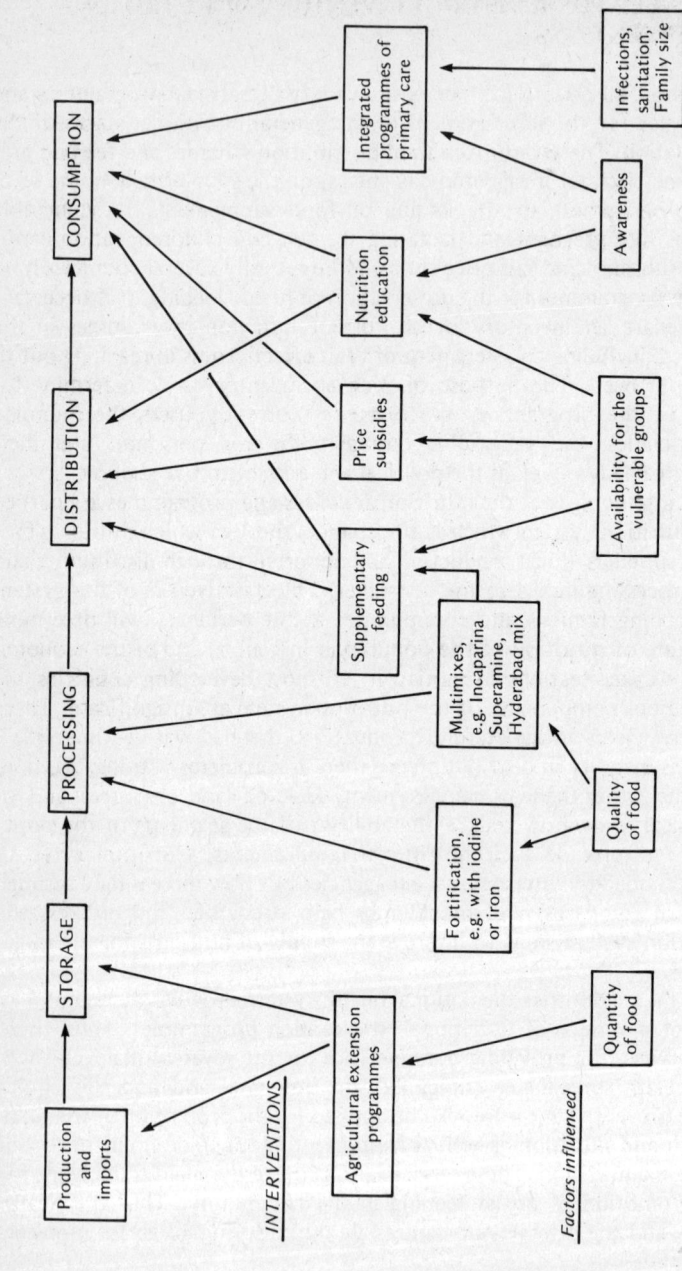

Figure 9.1 Nutrition interventions

ing the nutritional status of the vulnerable groups. The outreach clinics and home visiting further extend the scope of the health services into the home and remote communities. The impact of such direct interventions targeted at the family is strengthened by indirect preventive action for increasing the production and availability of food, improving the distribution system and purchasing power through local development activities, nutrition education and improved environmental and health conditions (figure 9.1). Such a multi-pronged approach addresses itself to the observation that nutrition problems are not solved through hand-outs of food, but require consideration of basic development tools like improved agricultural techniques; facilities for preservation, storage and transport; credit facilities; wages and prices policies; and educational programmes. Malnutrition is both a consequence as well as a contributory factor in underdevelopment. One needs to fight the prejudice that nutrition is social welfare. Instead, for the individual it is the foundation to good health and for the community, the cornerstone of development.

COVERAGE, A KEY ISSUE

However, a major factor in the success or otherwise of any programme is the coverage of the target groups. In developing countries lack of coverage has been identified as the main obstacle to the success of health and nutrition programmes. The recent successes in several countries with different political ideologies varying from China and Cuba to Sri Lanka, Kerala and Tanzania, are not due to any technical breakthroughs, but have been achieved by providing high coverage rates through a variety of means. In the district inventory a key question to ask will be with regard to the extent of coverage achieved. For each intervention being implemented in the district, the target population of beneficiaries needs to be defined and the proportion reached by the programme on a regular basis must be ascertained. For a large number of preventive actions, a measurable impact is usually found when a minimum of 80 per cent coverage of the target population is achieved.

ESTIMATING TARGET GROUPS

In measuring coverage it is best to work from periphery to the centre, or from bottom upwards as planners would say. It is reasonable to think of each village or hamlet as a distinct group and assess the coverage with nutrition programmes separately. The more geographically remote a community is from the centre, the greater the need for measuring coverage.

In all developing countries detailed demographic information is not available. The local branches of the political party, the agricultural department, the village leader or the school teacher may provide the number of families living in a given village. It is reasonable to assume a birth rate of between 35 and 40 per 1000 in order to estimate the number of *babies* born each year. When the number of infants under 1 year of age is known for a population group, it can be assumed that there are 10 per cent more *pregnant women* then there are infants. The number of *lactating women* can then be obtained by the formula

= No. of infants X Average duration of lactation in months ÷ 12.

Having obtained the approximate numbers in each target group, it is then possible to measure the availability and accessibility of services, the quality of care, the method of selection of beneficiaries and the criteria used for such a selection. It is obvious that the process of selection of the at-risk groups would be more effective if the coverage of the vulnerable groups is adequate. If the services reach only 20 per cent of the rural populations and the urban poor on a regular basis, then at-risk selection is occurring only amongst them, and the large majority of families derive only episodic benefit if any. This is at present the case in many developing countries and rapid expansion of coverage with basic health care is of the utmost importance.

THE NEED FOR INTEGRATION

Adequate food and nutrition is one of the five basic human needs, the others being adequate supplies of safe water and sanitation, basic health care, adequate shelter and basic education. Hence linkages between programmes are essential to ensure integrated development. Even though at the planning level there may be different ministries and governmental departments responsible for specific national programmes, at the level of the village and the home the impact should occur together and become mutually additive. This is especially so with regard to health and nutrition activities. Both are the expressions of multiple intertwined biological and social factors. The relationship between infection and undernutrition has been stressed in several of the preceding chapters. Similarly, the quantity and quality of water and sanitation determine the incidence of diarrhoea and intestinal helminths. The socioeconomic integration and development of the disadvantaged groups has been one major factor in the nutritional improvement in several countries. Because of the biological and social links between nutritional status, health status, living conditions, literacy and family size, it stands to reason that dealing with these areas simultaneously can achieve greater impact.

Hence the rationale for linking nutrition interventions with programmes of primary care.

INNOVATIVE APPROACHES

One major obstacle to achieving adequate coverage with primary health care is an inadequate health infrastructure. Though most countries include the construction of health centres and sub-centres as part of the national development programmes, the resources have not been enough, nor are they equitably and rationally distributed. Curative services still continue to take more than three-quarters of the national expenditure on health in many countries. Faced with the twin dilemma of inequity and disparities the district health team finds expansion of coverage an uphill struggle. Here innovative approaches in the form of auxiliaries and village health workers have been evolved and found to be remarkably successful. With adequate encouragement and support, these minimally trained workers are able to apply the main principles of health and good nutrition in remote rural homes. In this way they represent the distant arm of the health infrastructure. The second obstacle to full coverage with the conventional forms of health services has been the question of their acceptability to the traditional society. Here again the resistance of tradition is overcome when the providers of care are from amongst the community selected on the basis of their willingness to serve, and participating in the cultural and economic life of the community in which they are resident. The challenge to the district health team is not so much one of creating and training such a cadre of village health workers as that of successfully linking this popular arm of the system with the formal health service.

THE THREE TIERS IN THE ICEBERG OF MALNUTRITION

Clinically apparent malnutrition rests on the intensity and prevalence of infective illness. This is the second tier of the overall problem of malnutrition. The roles of infective illnesses like measles, whooping cough and respiratory as well as parasitic illnesses have been referred to in the preceding chapters. Diarrhoeal disease is another major contributory factor. Health activities of a non-nutritional nature like immunisation, oral rehydration at the village level, and facilities for early treatment of common illnesses as well as for child-spacing can have a major impact on the incidence of malnutrition. The services and approaches necessary for dealing with this second tier of the problem of malnutrition through primary care with adequate coverage as the main objective have been mentioned above. They are being developed in all countries in response to the call by the World Health Organisation for 'Health care for all by the year 2000'.

The third tier of the iceberg, and the main fountainhead of malnutrition, is the disadvantage of poverty. Poor nutrition is the result of a complex web of poverty and underdevelopment. Here poverty has a much broader meaning than simply low income or unavailability of land. It also means poor environment and housing, illiteracy, recurrent ill health, cultural deprivation, poor family relationships and increased risk of violence as well as mental illness and alcoholism in the family. In the average district of a developing country up to half the population may be living below the breadline, and in the urban squatter settlements the proportion may be even higher. How can the district health team address this complex problem of disadvantage, especially when there are so few models to follow, and in all professional training the subject is hardly ever discussed? Furthermore, in those countries which have succeeded in alleviating mass poverty the programmes and activities are underpinned by political ideologies. In many social groups poverty and oppression go hand in hand, and a highly conservative health profession has traditionally preferred to steer clear of this area.

Several guiding principles have been identified as a result of successful programmes of community health in many countries. It is the common experience that wherever social disparities exist, the benefits of services and intervention programmes are distributed in proportion to the disparity. Thus, the better-offs derive greater benefits than those lower down on the social pecking order. In the case of supplementary feeding programmes, for example, the truly needy families may derive no or little benefit. Hence it is essential to introduce safety devices that would divert the major thrust of the interventions towards the needy groups. Two well-tried methods are the use of village health workers and the village health committee. In the case of the *village health worker*, if the community elects one from amongst the upper social strata it may be useful to have an additional worker specifically for the lower socioeconomic class. The *village health committee* with adequate representation of disadvantaged groups has been found to be a powerful tool for the equitable distribution of information and agricultural resources like seeds, fertilisers and water. In rural communities where such social organisations do not exist, these benefits accrue only to the bigger landlords who are able to establish closer links with the appropriate officials. A third approach is through the creation of community awareness through regular dialogue which provides the psychological base for the community health programme. The objective here is to lead towards creating *social groups* through ongoing dialogue. These groups then become forums for discussions on specific problems facing the community and become care-takers of activities like literacy classes, sewing groups, parents' clubs, play-schools, farmer's clubs, youth clubs and so on. The underdeveloped community is usually the one with no social organisation. A social infra-structure provides the pegs and supports on which community activities hang together, besides generating community cohesion. Here again, if care is taken to include families from disadvantaged groups and the activities slanted towards their needs, the benefits of interventions at several levels can be made available to them. Health professionals are often conditioned by their training in predominantly curative medicine to look for a single quick-fix solution for community nutrition. It is therefore necessary to stress that in community health, including nutrition, all interventions can only be undertaken with people and through people. There is no other way. Hence the importance of creating several forums for mobilising community opinion. Nor has the professional all the answers. Such forums provide opportunities for learning from the experience of the people, and for devising ways and means of putting local experience to work and solve problems in consultation with community groups.

A STRATEGY OF 'NUTRITION WITH THE PEOPLE'

The above discussion on the three tiers of the iceberg of malnutrition and the possible intervention at the level of each tier enables us to evolve a total strategy for improving community nutrition. Clearly, those who are malnourished (second- and third-degree) require rehabilitation with or without prior hospitalisation. Those with mild-moderate malnutrition can be helped in the home through nutrition education of the parents, cooking demonstrations, food supplements and home visiting. The priority here is to channel nutritional resources to families with a nutritional disorder diagnosed in one of their members in order to tide them over a difficult period. At the same time the knowledge and skills of parents are being improved through demonstrations and education. Experience in several countries has shown that above the poverty threshold, malnutrition arises from faulty feeding practices, especially bottle feeding with powdered milk and formulae. Families who are in a position to reallocate 5 per cent of the total family caloric intake to the youngest child can prevent malnutrition through behaviour change as a result of nutrition education. Below the poverty threshold attempts to alleviate malnutrition through education alone will not be successful. Simultaneous increase in real income is necessary, though experience in Ghana, Upper Volta and Papua-New Guinea suggests that reduction in prevalence rates of malnutrition is possible through nutrition education and regular surveillance without any appreciable increase in real income. Nutrition education in the district must be uniform in order to avoid conflicting information being given, and should be simple. Experience in several countries suggests that the most effective way is to have specific and simplified 'messages' using the same phrases both through the mass media and through individual counselling.

However, the most important aspect of the strategy for the promotion of adequate nutrition will be regular surveillance so that minor problems can be dealt with on a day-to-day basis and individual counselling can be done as problems arise. Here the usefulness of surveillance services like the antenatal clinic and the under-5s clinics must be stressed. For these services to have an impact they must reach the maximum number on a regular basis even in a rudimentary form. In this respect the coverage target of a minimum of 80 per cent has already been mentioned, bearing in mind that the non-utilisers will be predominantly from amongst the groups who need the services most. They need to be included in the strategy of coverage by appropriate modifications in the services. The integration of nutrition interventions and surveillance services into a unified scheme is shown in Fig. 9.2.

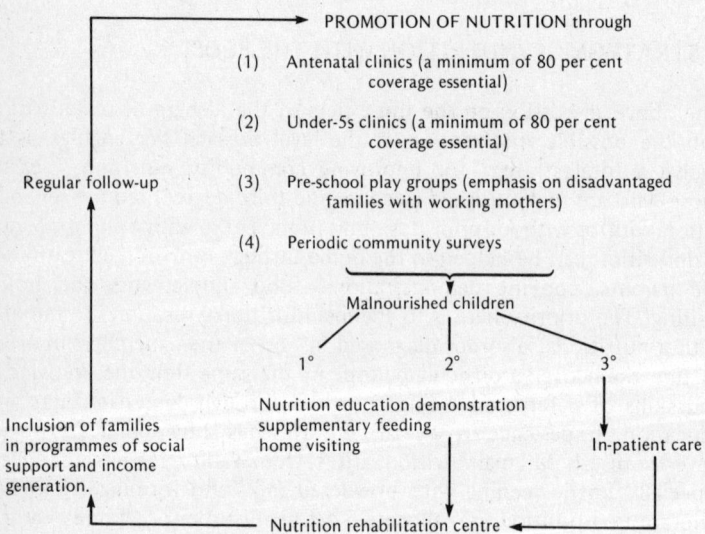

Figure 9.2 Integration of nutrition interventions and surveillance services

Regular coverage of vulnerable groups by the surveillance services of the district helps to identify those 'at risk' and thereby to anticipate problems. Here again the wider the coverage the more efficient is the 'at risk' selection. Those groups or families who do not make use of the services regularly may have a greater proportion of individuals at risk. Almost all countries use criteria for the selection of at-risk mothers and children. The objective always is to anticipate problems and have resources and solutions at hand to deal with them when they arise. Table 9.1 gives the more common criteria for selection.

Table 9.1 *Selection of 'at-risk' mothers and children*

At-risk mother	At-risk child
(1) Age below 15 and over 40	(1) Low birth weight.
(2) Height below 150 cm.	(2) Multiple pregnancy — twins, triplets, etc.
(3) First and after the fifth pregnancy.	(3) Birth order of 5 and above.
(4) Pre-pregnancy weight of less than 40 kg or weight gain of less than 7 kg in pregnancy.	(4) Pregnancy in the mother before the child is 18 months old.
(5) Previous history of still-birth, neonatal death or low birth weight.	(5) Absence of breast milk.
(6) Anaemia in pregnancy.	(6) Recent measles, whooping cough, diarrhoea or any major illness.
(7) Social problems like alcoholism or unemployment in the family.	(7) History of malnutrition or death in a sib.
(8) Abandoned mothers.	
(9) Socially deprived groups.	(8) Lack of weight gain in last 2 months.
(10) Short birth interval ($<$ 24 months).	(9) Social problems: (a) illegitimate child, one-parent family, abandoned child; (b) unemployment, chronic illness or alcoholism in parent; (c) socially deprived groups.

Services for health surveillance should be looked upon more as social services than strictly medical. Diagnosis of 'interesting' conditions is of secondary importance. Through continuing contact with a large

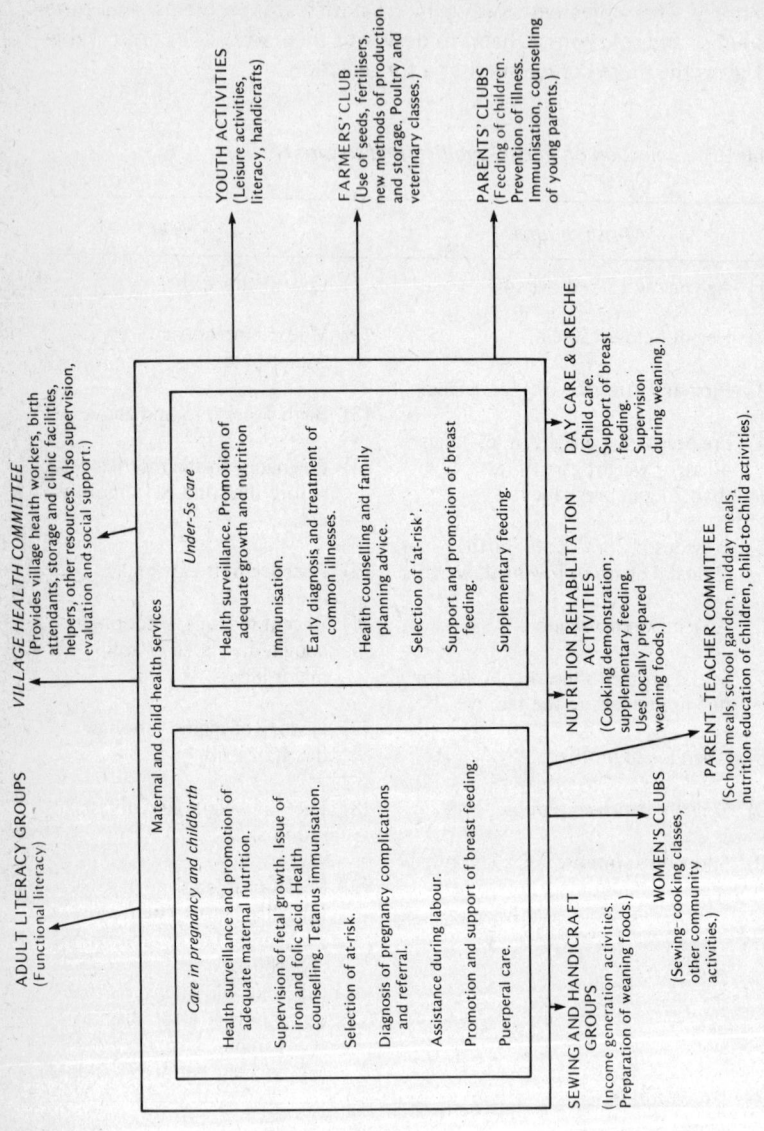

Figure 9.3 Interrelationships between health and nutrition interventions and community social groups

number of families such services help to build rapport with the community and provide a vital interface between the community and the medical services. They reach far out into the community compared to the health centre or the hospital. If the coverage is good their influence can be made to be felt in every rural home. Besides, the village health worker and the traditional birth attendant provide the distant arm of the maternal and child health services. In order to become truly community oriented the maternal and child health services need to work closely with the various social groups in the community. The activities of such groups then become complementary to the objectives of the services for mothers and children, by providing helpers and essential goods (like pre-packed medicines or locally prepared weaning foods). One major objective of health and nutrition interventions is to bring about change of behaviour and attitudes. This is not easy. In every human group acceptance of new ideas follows a bell-shaped (Gaussian) curve. Some of us, about 3 per cent, are innovators; about 12 per cent are early adopters of new ideas, and another 35 per cent are late adopters. Of the remainder, another 35 per cent are cautious followers and about 15 per cent are laggards. The various social groups in the community tend to attract the more forward-looking individuals (innovators and early adoptors) in the community and provide the opportunities and training ground for leadership. By creating such groups and establishing mutually supportive relationships with them the health services can prepare the ground for innovation.

A conceptual framework for the interrelationships between health services, nutrition interventions and the community social groups is provided in figure 9.3.

Active participation by disadvantaged families in all the above communal activities is essential. It is the only way of preventing alienation and creating community cohesion. In fact, several of the activities may provide entry points for the disadvantaged into the network of health and nutrition interventions. The disadvantaged are the ones carrying the triple burdens of social stigma, poverty and malnutrition together with ill-health. The large proportion of health and nutrition problems are amongst these social groups and all ways and means of drawing them into the fold of the community and social programmes must be explored.

URBAN AREAS

The urban poor present a major challenge in several ways. Firstly, the phenomenon of urban growth is new and there are virtually no models of service programmes that can be followed or adapted. Secondly, the increase in population has outstripped the rate at which the conventional and institutionalised services can be expanded. Finally, a major part of the increase represents overflow of rural poverty into the cities, so that there is an influx into the cities of people with virtually no skills and resources to enable them to participate in the economic life of the modern urban sector. In the year 1970 there were 79 cities with populations over the million mark in the developing world. By the year 1985 it is estimated that there will be 147 such cities. The ripples of this process are felt in every small district town. Even though absolute numbers may not be increasing at the same rate as in the capital cities, it is important to bear in mind that the resources at the district centres are much less compared to those in the capital cities. Complacency may allow the problem to get out of hand.

It has been estimated that up to a third of the population of many cities may be living in slums or squatter settlements, and a quarter to a half of the families live in states of intense deprivation. Unemployment rates vary from 10 to 40 per cent in various surveys. Food intake of the urban squatter population is frequently, though not always, less than in rural areas. This also holds true for intake of several nutrients besides calories.

New arrivals in the city are affected in a variety of ways. They step out of the social and cultural milieu of the rural society and into the anonymity of an exploiting city. Whatever social and cultural support they had in village life is now left behind, and psychological illness or depression is a common phenomenon. In the teeming slum there is no home garden or livestock, and no way in which foods purchased in the market can be supplemented with those produced at home. Most new arrivals, particularly if they are from a different region of the country, often find strange new foods. Choice must be made among these unfamiliar foods. In the absence of nutrition education, traditional foods are discarded in favour of cheaper or convenience foods. This is especially so when such foods are being seductively advertised, as in the case of powdered milks and other infant foods.

In many countries a number of national nutrition programmes have been formulated and these are mainly directed at the urban populations. Nine types of direct nutrition interventions are in operation either singly or in various combinations in several countries. These are nutrition education; on-site or take-home feeding; provision of nutrient-dense foods (e.g. incaparina, superamine, faffa, bienestarina, bal-ahar, nutripak, Hyderabad-mix etc.); ration shops; food coupons; food fortification (e.g. with iodine); direct nutrient dosage (e.g. with vitamin A); food processing; and distribution (e.g. enriched wheat flour). The major deficiencies have been inconsistent supplies and inadequate coverage.

Provision of basic health care to the urban poor is as scanty as in rural areas in spite of their comparative proximity to hospitals and other health facilities. This is partly because urban settlements tend to spring up overnight. Many have highly mobile populations. The social disparities between the providers of care and the beneficiaries are even greater in cities than in rural areas, and the use of outreach services, auxiliaries, part-time health workers and birth attendants has not been adequately explored for urban populations. An urgent need is for the rapid deployment of programmes of maternal and child health to the urban poor so as to provide the framework for health and nutrition interventions. The rural model as described above can be adapted for the urban areas utilising community institutions like schools, neighbourhood health centres, community centres and clubs all supported by neighbourhood groups and institutions.

FURTHER READING

Harvard Institute for International Development. *Nutrition Intervention in Developing Countries,* vols. I-V. Delgeschlager, Gunn & Hain, Cambridge, Mass., 1981.

Mayer, J. and Dwyer, J. *Food and Nutrition Policy in a Changing World.* Oxford University Press, New York, 1979.

Index

Adaptive changes, in malnutrition, 106-8
Agricultural technology, 5
Amino acids
    comparison of patterns in human and cow's milk with egg, 56
    in foods, 25, 29
Anaemia, 167-81
    accompanying malnutrition, 116-17
    and intestinal helminths, 179-81
    etiological factors, 170-81
    in children, 168-70
    in tropical splenomegaly syndrome, 181
    megaloblastic, 176
    prevalence of, 167-70
    related to cultural practices, 180
Antibodies in human milk, 73
Artificial feeding
    dangers of, 66-9
    economic aspects of, 68
    hypernatraemia, 68
    metabolic acidosis, 68
At-risk selection, 191

Balanced diet, preparation of, 28-32
β-carotene, 136-9
Beliefs, related to foods, 9-11
Beri-Beri, 160-1
Birthweight, 36
    and foetal body composition, 48
    effects of nutritional deficiency in pregnancy, 44-7
Blood loss, 180
Breast feeding, 54-82
    intervention programmes for promotion of, 78-81
Breast milk, *see* Human milk

Calcium
    food sources of, 148
    intake of, 147-8
Carbohydrates
    in human milk, 62-3
    in tropical foods, 17-25
    metabolism of, in malnutrition, 121
Cellular content of human milk, 75
Cereals, 16-24
    Maize, 22-4
    Rice, 20-2
    Sorghum, 24
    Wheat, 17-20
Child spacing, 77-8
Classification
    Gomez, 109
    of malnutrition, 105-13
    Wellcome, 108-9
Co-enzymes, 152
Community
    constructing nutritional profile of, 130
    making a diagnosis of malnutrition, 129-32
    monitoring nutrition of, 128-9
    nutrition intervention based on, 127-8
    nutrition with people, strategy of, 189-93
    programmes for better nutrition, 182-95

Index

Community-centred approaches in malnutrition, 127-8
Coverage, 185
Cultural practices, 7-11
 and anaemia, 180
 for weaning, 86-8

Defence mechanisms and malnutrition, 122-3
Definition of malnutrition, 105-13
7-dehydrocholesterol, 145
Diets for weaning and energy intake, 88-9

Edible oil plants, 26-7
Electrolytes, in human and cow's milk, 66-8
Endocrinological changes in pregnancy, 34
Environment, 1-3
 systems of interaction with, 4-14
Epidemiology
 of protein-energy malnutrition, 104-5
 of rickets, 141-4
 of xerophthalmia, 135-7

Fats
 composition of, 58
 content in cow's and human milk, 59-61
 in common tropical foods, 26-7
 in milk, 58-60
 metabolism of, in malnutrition, 121
Female stature, 35
Foetus
 and size of the mother, 35
 birth weight, 36
 body composition of, 48
 cellular growth, 47-8
 growth of, 34-53
 nutritional requirement of, 37-8
Folic acid, 176-9
 absorption of, 177-8
 megaloblastic anaemia, 176-7
 physiological role of, 176
 requirements in infants, 179
 requirements in pregnancy, 178
 source of, 177
Food industry, 14-15
Food processing, home, 13-14
Food storage, 11-13

Gastrointestinal tract, in malnutrition, 118-19
Gomez classification, 108-9
Growth
 catch-up, 91-2
 effects of infections on, 90-1
 effects of malnutrition on, 106-12
 failure of, in malnutrition, 113
 longitudinal studies of, 92-6

Haemopoietic system, changes in malnutrition, 119
Health profession, role of, in promoting breast feeding, 79-80
Health system, as outlet for nutrition interventions, 183
Heart, changes in malnutrition, 119
Human milk, 55-78
 acid load in, 68
 amino-acid pattern of, 55-7, 64
 and child spacing, 77-8
 and mother-infant bonding, 77
 antibodies in, 73
 as a biological mediator, 76-7
 as a nutrient, 63-6
 as a protective agent, 69-75
 carbohydrate in, 62-3
 cellular content of, 75
 cellular mechanisms of synthesis and secretion of, 64-6
 electrolyte content of, 66-8
 fat composition of, 58-62
 for low birth weight infants, 83-4
 immunoglobulins in, 70-3
 intervention programmes for promotion of, 78-81
 lactoferrin in, 73-4
 metabolism of protein, 57
 other protective factors, 75-6
Hypercalcaemia, 149
Hypernatraemia, 68

Immunoglobulins in human milk, 70–3
Infancy
  anaemia in, 168–70, 175–6
  body iron, 175
  cord blood haemoglobin, 175
  energy intake, 83
  essential amino acids, requirements of, 55
  estimated intakes of nutrients, 56
  folic acid and B_{12} requirements, 179
  intake of fat and growth of nervous system, 59–61
  metabolism of milk proteins in, 57
  protein requirements in, 54–7
Infection, role of, in malnutrition, 90–1, 96–8
Innovative approaches, 187
Integration of programmes, 186–7, 190, 193
Intervention programmes
  community-centred approaches in malnutrition, 127–8
  coverage, 185
  for improved community nutrition, 182–95
  for prevention of rickets, 150–1
  for prevention of xerophthalmia, 139–41
  for promotion of breast feeding, 78–81
  for protection of the weanling, 99–103
  for provision of health care, 102–3
  for reduction of bulk in diet, 100
  health system as outlet for, 183
  in pregnancy, 50–3
  in the district, inventory of, 183–5
  in urban areas, 193–5
  monitoring community nutrition, 128–32
  policies for production of multimixes, 99–100
  target groups, 185–6
Intestinal helminths and anaemia, 180
Intestine, in malnutrition, 98–9
Iron, 170–6
  daily turnover of, 173–4
  in normal infant, 175
  physiology of absorption, 171–3
  sources of, 170–1

Kwashiorkor, 106
  clinical features of, 113–22

La Leche League, 79
Lactoferrin in human milk, 73–4
Land tenure, 6
Legumes, 25–6
  amino acids in, 25
Liver, changes in kwashiorkor, 117
Longitudinal studies
  Gambia, 94
  Guatemala, 94–5
  India, 92
  main findings, 95–6
  Mexico, 96
  of child growth, 92–6
  Uganda, 93

Maize, 3, 22–4
Malaria
  anaemia in infants, 180–1
  haemolytic anaemia in pregnancy, 180
  placental infection, 40
Malnutrition
  adaptive changes in, 106–8
  and the brain, 120–1
  and the weaning period, 83–103
  changes in digestive system, 117–19
  effects on haemopoietic system, 119
  effects on the heart, 119
  gut dynamics in, 98–9
  management of, 123–5
  metabolic changes in, 121–2
  mild-moderate, 106–13
  protein-energy, 104–33
  role of infection, 90–1, 96–8

the muscle compartment in, 119–20
three tiers of, 187–9
Marasmus, 106, 115
Measuring malnutrition, 106–12
Medical practices interfering with lactation, 80
Metabolic response in infection, 96–7
Mild and milk products, 27
  carbohydrate in, 62–3
  electrolytes in cow's and human milk, 66–8
  fat composition in human and cow's milk, 58–62
  metabolism of milk protein in infants, 57
Minerals in tropical foods, 29
Mortality
  pre-school, and malnutrition, 105
  risks in malnutrition, 112–13
Mother-infant bonding, 77
Multi-mixes, 28
Muscle, changes in malnutrition, 119–20

NapCal per cent, 30–2, 100, 101
Nervous system, effects of malnutrition, 120–1
Niacin (nicotinamide), 153–8
  pellagra, 154–8
  physiological role of, 154
  sources of, 153
  tryptophan, 153
Nutrition rehabilitation centres, 125–6
Nutrition system, 183
Nutritional anaemia, 167–81
  and intestinal helminths, 179–81
  etiological factors, 170–81
  hypochromic, 171–3
  in children, 168–70
  megaloblastic, 176
  prevalence of, 167–70
Nutritional status of mother and foetal growth, 35–6

Oedema, 113
Osteomalacia, 148–9

Pancreas, in kwashiorkor, 118
Pellagra, 154–8
  clinical features of, 156
  prevention, 158
  treatment, 158
Physiology
  in protein-energy malnutrition, 117–22
  of daily turnover of iron, 173–4
  of iron absorption, 171–3
  of niacin (nicotinic acid), 154
  of pyridoxine, 163
  of riboflavin, 162
  of Vitamin A, 137–9
  of Vitamin D, 144–7
  of vitamins of B group, 151–3
Placenta
  mechanisms of transfer, 39
  the role of, 38–40
  transfer of iron, 175
Poverty, 188
Pregnancy
  effects of nutritional deficiency, 44–7
  effects of supplementation, 49–50
  endocrinological changes in, 34
  intervention programmes, 50–3
  iron and folic acid requirements in, 42–3, 175, 178
  malaria in, 40, 180
  nutrition in, 34–53
  recommended allowances, 43–4
  weight gain in, 41–2
Pre-term infant, feeding of, 83–4
Prevalence
  of anaemia, 167–70
  of malnutrition, 104
Protective factors in human milk, 69–75
Protein
  content of tropical foods, 29
  quality of, 28
  metabolism of, in malnutrition, 121–22

requirements in infancy, 54–7
reference, 28
score, 30
Protein–energy malnutrition, 104–33
   adaptive changes in, 106–8
   arm circumference in, 111–12
   associated deficiencies in, 115–17
   classification, 105–13
   clinical features of, 113–22
   complications of, 124
   innovative approaches in management, 125–7
   management of, 123–5
   metabolic changes in, 117–22
   monitoring community nutrition, 128–32
   pathological features of, 117–22
   weight charts in, 109–10
Pyridoxine, 163

Riboflavine, 161–3
   physiological role of, 162
   sources of, 162
Rice, 3, 20–2
   nutrient losses in washing, 21
   nutritional value, 22
Rickets, 116, 141–51
   clinical manifestations of, 149–50
   in temperate climates, 143–4
   in the tropics, 144
   prevention of, 150–1
   treatment of, 150
Rural poor, 6

Small-for-dates infant, feeding of, 84–5
Social class and birth weight, 36
Social groups, 192–3
Social systems, 6–7
Sorghum, 24
Strategy of community nutrition, 189–93
Stunting, 106–7

Target groups, 185–6

Thiamine, 159–61
   anti-thiamine factors, 159–60
   Beri-beri, 160–1
   sources of, 159
Treatment of malnutrition, 123–5
   in hospital, 124
   in the home, 125
Tropical foods, 16–33
   nutrients in, 29
Tropical splenomegaly syndrome, 181
Tubers, 24–5
   cassava, 24
   plantains, 24–5
   potato, 25

Under-5s clinic, 102
Urban areas, 193–5
Urbanisation and malnutrition, 108

Village health workers, 102
Vitamin A, 134–41
   physiology of, 137–9
Vitamin B_{12}, 176–9
   absorption of, 177–8
   megaloblastic anaemia, 176–7
   physiological role of, 176
   requirements in infants, 179
   requirements in pregnancy, 178
   sources of, 177
Vitamin D, 141–51
   physiology of, 144–7
   sources of, 145
Vitamins, in tropical foods, 29
Vitamins of the B group, 151–65
   B_{12}, 176–9
   deficiency of, 116, 152
   errors of metabolism responsive to, 164
   folic acid, 176–9
   pellagra, 154–8
   physiological role of, 151
   pyridoxine, 163
   riboflavine, 161–3
   thiamine, 159–61

Wasting, 106–7
Weaning period, 83–103
   dangers of, 86–8

intercurrent infections, 90-1
Weanling, appetite and food intake, 89
Weight charts, 109-10
Wellcome classification, 108-9
Wheat, 3, 17-20
    bread, nutrient content of, 20
    chapatti, nutrient content of, 20
    flour, composition of, 19

Xerophthalmia, 115, 134-41
    epidemiology of, 135-7
    prevention of, 139-41